THERAPEUTIC RECREATION SERVICE

THERAPEUTIC RECREATION SERVICE

An Applied Behavioral Science Approach

ELLIOTT M. AVEDON
University of Waterloo, Ontario

Prentice-Hall, Inc., *Englewood Cliffs, New Jersey*

Library of Congress Cataloging in Publication Data

Avedon, Elliott M
   Therapeutic recreation service.

   Includes bibliographical references.
   1. Recreational therapy.   I. Title.
[DNLM: 1. Occupational therapy. 2. Recreation.
3. Social behavior. WM450 A948t 1974]
RC489.R4A9   615'.8515   73-13903
ISBN 0-13-914879-5

©1974 by Prentice-Hall, Inc., Englewood Cliffs, New Jersey. All rights reserved. No part of this book may be reproduced in any form or by any means without permission in writing from the publisher. Printed in the United States of America.

10 9 8 7 6 5 4 3

Prentice-Hall International, Inc., *London*
Prentice-Hall of Australia, Pty, Ltd., *Sydney*
Prentice-Hall of Canada, Ltd., *Toronto*
Prentice-Hall of India Private Limited, *New Delhi*
Prentice-Hall of Japan, Inc., *Tokyo*

To my wife and children,
who alternately badgered me and pampered me
so this book might be written.

Contents

	Preface	ix
SECTION I	**INTRODUCTION**	**1**
1	Historical Precedents	4
2	The Immediate Past	12
3	Principles That Influence Service	18
4	Some Kindred Services	28
SECTION II	**THE KNOWLEDGE AND SKILL BASE FOR SERVICE**	**41**
5	Aspects of Recreation	43
6	Elements of Service—Part I	54
7	Elements of Service—Part II	80

SECTION III SOCIAL AND BEHAVIORAL FACTORS IN PROGRAMMING — 105

8   *Social and Behavioral Factors in Program Development*   *106*

9   *Application of Systems Analysis Procedures to Program Planning in Therapeutic Recreation Service by Carol A. Peterson*   *128*

10   *Social and Behavioral Factors in Program Organization*   *156*

11   *Social and Behavioral Factors in Program Content*   *173*

12   *Aspects of Professional Practice*   *215*

Index   *235*

Preface

The provision of service to persons who are limited in some manner preventing them from taking advantage of the range of experiences available today for recreation is not the province of any one group of persons. It is the concern of many people running the gamut from the parent of a child with disability, to the administrator of a home for aging persons, to the parole officer responsible for delinquent adolescents. However, just as all things in contemporary society have become more complex, it has become apparent to these persons that the provision of recreation service is no longer a simple matter, and requires the acquisition of a number of inter-related knowledges, abilities, and skills.

When I was an undergraduate, a range of educational experiences dealing with "recreation leadership" were available. However, most of these dealt with the what, how, and who of practice, with little information presented about the "why." It was expected that the student learn about "why" in other courses and apply these learnings to recreation practice. If you were lucky, you had an effective field work supervisor who helped you make this type of application.

The amount of knowledge relating to "why" has increased considerably since I was an undergraduate. It is common practice today to incorporate knowledges from the behavioral and social sciences in courses concerning "recreation leadership," but it is difficult to put these together in an applied fashion so they are meaningful and practical.

That is the intent of this book—to draw from the behavior and social sciences, those aspects of their knowledge base which have relevance for the practice of therapeutic recreation service.

After a brief excursion into the historical roots of practice, and a mini view of contemporary developments, a philosophical rationale for practice is offered. Through the years, I have found considerable concurrance with this point of view, but must admit that some of my colleagues continue to take issue with certain aspects of this rationale.

Because of the inter-relatedness of various "helping professions" and the role of diffusion caused by the multiple use of popular recreation media, I have attempted to unravel this professional tangle through the presentation in Chapter 4 of parallel factors concerning these professions.

The heart of the text begins in Section II with an examination of required knowledges and skills for application in practice. After putting the phenomena of recreation in perspective, the elements of therapeutic recreation service are explored.

A detailed look at programming from a social and behavioral point of view appears in Section III. In this section, I have applied knowledge from various disciplines to program planning, program organization, and program content.

Throughout the text, I have used actual case material from practice to illustrate various theoretical notions. This material has been altered somewhat to protect the anonymity of the persons and settings involved. At times a number of actual situations have been fused together into a prototype situation. The final chapter offers the reader an opportunity to apply material contained in this book to practice, as well as to apply learnings from other sources.

Many of my colleagues and former students have contributed to the writing of this book. Drs. Carol A. Peterson and Fred W. Martin have permitted the use of original material relating to their special competences. The latter also deserves my thanks for reviewing various sections of the manuscript, and making helpful suggestions or raising significant questions. Others have sent case records from their own practice for my use. Much of the selection of the material to be included is a consequence of the endless probing and discussions with my students and colleagues during the past decade. Thanks for the interaction diagrams in Chapter 10 go to Mr. William Barton who out of frustration with my art work at the blackboard a number of years ago, formalized my sketches into the present charts. Finally a special note of appreciation is due to my friend and colleague, Dr. Richard G. Kraus, who steadfastly encouraged the writing of this book.

To my colleagues in the Faculty of Human Kinetics and Leisure Studies and to the staff of the Computer Center of the University of Waterloo go my thanks for their patience and assistance.

E.M.A.
Waterloo, Ontario

THERAPEUTIC RECREATION SERVICE

I
INTRODUCTION

Recreation is one of those special aspects of civilization which has the potential to contribute to the sustaining of life, the prevention of dysfunction, and the treatment of pathology. With regard to recreation's potential contribution to the sustaining of life, the Spanish poet Cervantes wrote:

> The bow cannot always stand bent, nor can human frailty subsist without some recreation.[1]

Cervantes suggests that recreation has a sustaining value for the human spirit, a value that is easily understood in the context of contemporary society. Recreation is one of the few remaining avenues in modern society that offers an opportunity to do something we want to do when we want to do it, at our own tempo and speed—to precisely the degree of involvement that is most satisfying to us. Recreation makes possible the gratification of certain personal needs which we cannot fulfill in other ways because of the everyday demands placed upon us by employment, family obligations, and social responsibility.

One explanation of how recreation sustains each of us was offered by Haun. He indicated that recreation is

> man's sovereign opportunity to tap life's deepest currents; to have again and again the vital experience of integration in which all his levers and gears and shafts and wheels mesh in perfect synchronization with the world of people and of matter; to feel again and again the happy power of

[1] Miguel de Cervantes (1547-1616), *Don Quixote*, I Book 4, line 21.

facility where impulse, performance, and result blend uninterruptedly into a unified whole.[2]

Society has long been aware of what happens to a person when he is denied opportunities for this experience. As evidence, we note this remarkable psychodynamic picture presented by Shakespeare:

> Sweet recreation barred, what doth ensue / But moody moping, and dull melancholy, / Kinsman to grim and comfortless despair, / And at her heels a huge infectious troop / Of pale distemperatures and foes of life.[3]

As a consequence, society has sanctified the "work-play-Jack" philosophy, assuring a variety of recreations for both children and adults, so that Jack should not become moody, or mope, or suffer from dull melancholy and grim despair. It is interesting that sanctification has been extended over the years to include opportunities for the military at war, prisoners in correctional institutions, religious personnel in convents and monasteries, persons who reside in residential institutions such as hospitals, sanitoria, special schools, and other enclosed settings.

In addition to recreation in a preventive context, mankind also became consciously aware of recreation's remedial potential. This recognition must be very old, because evidence of the casual acceptance of this notion can be found in the following reported example of a man who, suffering from a reactive depression with suicidal tendencies, was "cured" by a recreative experience:

> at times an evil spirit from the Lord would seize him suddenly. His servants said to him, "You see, sir, how an evil spirit from God seizes you; why do you not command your servants here to go and find some man who can play the harp?—then, when the evil spirit from God comes on you, he can play and you will recover..." David came to Saul and entered his service... And whenever a spirit from God came upon Saul, David would take his harp and play on it, so that Saul found relief; he recovered and the evil spirit left him alone.[4]

The concept of *Therapeutic Recreation Service* is an outgrowth of (1) society's use of recreation to prevent dysfunction which results from a lack of opportunities for recreative experience among special groups of the population; and (2) the use of traditional recreation activity in the treatment of illness and disability. Although the concept has its roots in antiquity (as demonstrated in Chapter I), the genesis of the contemporary concept was in the United States, Canada, and Western Europe, the industrialized nations of the world.

This section includes a brief historical overview of the use of recreation first as a service within treatment-oriented institutions, and later to persons in

---

[2] Paul Haun, Recreation: *A Medical Viewpoint,* E. M. Avedon and F. B. Arje, eds. (New York: Teachers College Press, 1965), p. 37.
[3] William Shakespeare (1564-1616), *The Comedy of Errors,* act 5, sc. 1, lines 78-82.
[4] The New English Bible, 1 Sam. 16:14-23.

Introduction 3

noninstitutional settings. Information about some groups and major personalities who have influenced the development of the concept is also included.

The philosophical principles upon which service is based and the frame of reference within which service is offered, as well as a delineation of therapeutic recreation service from other types of service offered to the public, is presented in the latter chapter of the section. Although an attempt has been made to include a range of historical information, the reader is asked to view this section as illustrative, for a definitive history indicating the many roots and influences upon practice has yet to be written.

1
Historical Precedents

Ancient Civilizations

What is known of recreation and of illness during ancient times? What evidence is there that ancient peoples engaged in activities we identify as recreation? Among historians and archaeologists who study our heritage, there is often controversy over an artifact that has been found when there is no conclusive proof of how it was used in an ancient culture. This is usually true when something resembling a game board is found and dated in the second or third millennium, but it is equally true of Middle-American structures resembling ball courts that are approximately a thousand years old.

One scholar will say that the artifact was used for recreative purposes, while another will claim that it had a ritualistic or religious function in a given culture, and still a third will theorize that it served both functions. Sometimes one or the other theory will prove to be correct with the help of the translation of an inscription or the finding of a tomb painting or a painted pottery fragment depicting the use of the artifact.

From such findings, we know something of the daily lives of people who lived in such places as Babylon, Lagash, Nineveh, Jericho, and Ur. We have learned that they made music and they danced; they sang songs and they juggled; they entertained and they were entertained by professional entertainers. They had table games, gambling games, children's toys; they engaged in sports, festivals, and a host of other activities we identify as "recreation." We also know that there was public awareness of a variety of illnesses and disabilities, and an organized system to treat illness. There were even legal codes specifying penalties for medical malpractice.

Historical Precedents

Some of the evidence suggests that people of these cultures believed that illness and dysfunction was attributable to demons, evil spirits, and transgressions against the gods. Thus, care and treatment programs were in the hands of priests in most of the Fertile Crescent area. There are no specific records, written or otherwise, to prove that recreative experiences were provided in these cultures to prevent illness; however, there is ample evidence to indicate that many activities of a ritual nature (which we identify with recreation) were seasonally engaged in to propitiate the gods.

In ancient Egypt, priests established temples that were elaborate retreats used to treat the sick. Treatment prescribed by the priests consisted of rituals designed to appease the gods. The patients

> were required to walk in the beautiful gardens which surrounded the temples, or to row on the majestic Nile. Delightful excursions were planned for them under the plea of pilgrimages. Dances, concerts, and comic representations occupied a part of the day, as constituting the symbolic worship of some divinity.[1]

Although there are no comparable records, it was probably true that a convalescent sick person amused himself with an ancient counterpart of a jigsaw puzzle, or played a table game or two with another sick person or a member of his family. Game boards have been found that were cut into the roofing slabs of ancient Egyptian temples by workmen, who probably played these games during their "breaks", while the temple was being constructed. The Biblical extract quoted in the introduction is yet additional evidence of early use of recreative experience as treatment. However, we can only speculate at this time as to the extent of its conscious and deliberate use to prevent dysfunction and treat illness in these early civilizations.

Greece and Rome

The Greeks were among the first ancient people to consider medicine a nonreligious art, although they still attributed some illness to the gods. Greek physicians came from the laity rather than the priesthood. According to legend, the first Greek physician, Melampus, treated the daughters of Proteus by having them play a game that involved running. This is reported to have cured them of the delusion that they were cows.

Melampus taught Chiron, who in turn taught Aesculapius, the legendary physician who became the god of healing. Followers of Aesculapius built a number of temples that served as curative centers for the sick. The most famous of these, at Epidaurus, was built on the site of a primitive sanctuary, and was constantly improved during the first millennium. The temple was a cluster of facilities which included a library, a stadium, a theater, and a sanatorium that housed patients who came from all over the civilized world for "treatment." The

[1] W. A. F., Browne, *What Asylums Were, Are, and Ought To Be* (Edinburgh and London: Adam and Charles Black, 1837), pp. 141-42.

temple also served as the center for a variety of religious activities. Athletic contests were held here nine days after the Isthmian Games every four years. Plato wrote of the dramatic productions that were staged in the theater, and described the poetry and miming contests that were annual events. As in earlier cultures, many of these activities were first engaged in for religious reasons and later for their own sake. In fact, the English word "athlete" comes from the time after the golden age of Greece when participants in the Olympic games were no longer involved in the games for the glory of the gods but rather for the *athlon*—the prize they would win.

In ancient Greece, each school of philosophical thought contributed to the notion of how to live in order to prevent dysfunction and what to do if one became ill. For example, the mathematician Pythagoras also taught the healing art. For treatment of mental disorders, he urged the use of music in conjunction with gymnastics and dancing.

Roman warriors returned to Rome with new ideas and systems that had been prevalent among the peoples they conquered. As in the case of the Greeks, the religion of the Romans had little influence upon medical practice, so Roman practitioners were free to adopt foreign ideas quickly. Aesclepiades of Bithynia, a Greek physician practicing in Rome, felt that treatment of the mentally ill should be more humane, and thus in 124 A.D. he ordered that those in his charge be taken from their dark cells and brought out into the sunshine. He then provided music and song as well as gentle exercise for them. Another Roman physician, Soranus (98-138 A.D.), extolled the efficacy of music as a remedy for sciatica. He indicated that music charmed away the pain. Galen (130-201 A.D.), the last of the great ancient physicians, wrote that games that afford relaxation to the mind and body are best. For persons who were particularly disturbed and rather violent, he had a system of cure using music and poetry.

Both the Greeks and the Romans offered many activities under public auspices to prevent social dysfunction. The Greeks concentrated on resources for physical activity that would prevent the "disuse atrophy syndrome." In their writings they heralded the virtues of diet and exercise. However, not only were they concerned with physical activity as a tonic for the body, but they taught that intellectual activity was necessary as balance. In contrast, the Romans seemed less concerned with individual participation and envisioned the circus and other spectator activities as means of preventing social disorganization.

Roman medicine and health practices were the foundation for most of the practices carried on in Europe during the Middle Ages. However, there were also some early influences upon Europe from the Middle East and the Orient.

China and India

Sketchy records of ancient China refer to a great surgeon, Hua T'o (ca. 190 A.D.). San Kuo Chih has preserved this vignette, which indicates the skill of Hua T'o and offers an example of the use of a recreation that is quite rare today:

Historical Precedents

> Kuan Yu had no armour on . . . an arrow struck him in the arm . . . the head had been poisoned. The wound was deep, and the poison penetrated to the bone. The right arm was discoloured and swollen and useless. . . . Seeing that their leader would not retire and the wound showed no signs of healing, the various captains enquired far and near for a good surgeon to attend their general. One day a person arrived. . . . In his hand he carried a small black bag. He said his name was Hua T'o. . . . He had heard of the wound sustained by the famous hero and had come to heal it. . . . He found him engaged in a game of *wei-chi* [a table game of position and allignment using black and white counters on a marked board—the Japanese game of "GO"], although his arm was very painful. . . . Hua T'o was shown the injured arm. "There is some blackhead poison in the wound and it has penetrated to the bone. Unless the wound is soon treated the arm will become useless. . . . This is what I shall do. In a private room I shall erect a post with a ring attached. I shall ask you, Sir, to insert your arm in the ring, and I shall cover your head with a quilt so that you cannot see, and with a scalpel I shall open up the flesh right down to the bone. Then I shall scrape away the poison. This done, I shall dress the wound with a certain preparation, sew it up with a thread, and there will be no further trouble. But I think you may quail at the serverity of the treatment." Kuan Yu smiled, "It sounds easy enough, but why the post and ring?" Refreshments were then served, and after a few cups of wine the warrior extended his arm for the operation. With his other hand he went on with his game. Meanwhile the surgeon prepared his knife and called a lad to hold a basin beneath the limb. "I am just going to cut; do not start," said Hua T'o. . . . The surgeon then performed the operation as he had predescribed. . . . and all those near covered their eyes and turned pale. But Kuan Yu went on with his game, only drinking a cup of wine now and again. . . . When the wound had been cleansed, sewn up and dressed, the patient stood up smiling and said, "This arm is now as good as it ever was; there is no pain. Indeed, Master Leech, you are a marvel."[2]

Another famous method of Hua T'o was what he called "The Sport of Five Animals," which he recommended for those who engage in sedentary activity during the day, or for older persons who were no longer kept physically active. He wrote:

> The human body needs work, but it must not work to its utmost capacity. When it is in motion, the food is digested, and the blood circulates through the arteries in all directions, so that no disease can appear. Hence it is that the immortals of ancient days, while performing the inhalation process, and passing their time as dormant bears, looking around about like owls, twitched and stretched their loins and limbs, and moved their navel gates and their joints in order to hinder the advance of age. I have an art called the sport of five animals, namely, the tiger, the stag, the bear, the monkey, and the bird, by which illness can be cured,

---

[2] San Kuo Chih, *Romance of the Three Kingdoms,* Vol. II, trans. C. H. Brewitt Taylor (Shanghai, 1929), 156-59.

and which is good for the movements of the feet, when they accompany the process of inhalation. Whenever you feel unwell, stand up and imitate the movements of one of these animals; when you feel more comfortable and in a perspiration, put rice powder over your body, and you will presently feel quite nimble and well, and have a good a appetite.[3]

These two selections exemplify the Chinese use of activity in the treatment and prevention of illness. Although the basic theories of medicine differed from Western thought, the use of activity in the second selection does not markedly differ.

About the same time in India, a famous physician named Charaka was practicing in the province of Kashmir. As in the West, the concept of the hospital had taken hold in India, and Charaka wrote of the management of hospitalized patients.

It is no surprise that Charaka advocated the use of toys and games for patients in hospitals, because India was the birthplace of many popular recreative devices we use today: for example, chess, parchisi, backgammon, and dice. The Vedic literature includes a "Dice Song," telling of the trials and tribulations of the dice player. Toys and games were a natural aspect of Indian life at the time, and one would expect to find them everywhere, particularly in a hospital where people had time to use them. What is rather surprising, because it is still somewhat of an issue in a number of places today, is that Charaka felt that it was the responsibility of the hospital to supply the toys and games for patient use![4]

The Middle East

There is much in the literature to indicate that both Jewish and Moslem physicians of the early Middle Ages were more sophisticated than their European counterparts. For example, in a book written by Avicenna (980-1037 A.D.), a Persian physician, there is a discussion of the effect of water supply, climate, the seasons, bathing, sleep, and emotional disturbance upon health. He also discusses the therapeutic use of music in one chapter, and the care of aging persons in another.[5]

Nor is the level of sophistication limited to the literature. The following is a description of the Mansur Hospital at Cairo, which was completed and operating in the year 1284 A.D. There were

> male and female wards for general cases, also wards reserved for wounds, for eye diseases, and for fevers, the last mentioned being cooled by fountains. There were courtyards for lecturers, a botanical garden, a

---

[3] "Biography of Hua T'o," in *History of the Later Han,* cited by E. H. Hume, *The Chinese Way in Medicine* (Baltimore: The Johns Hopkins Press, 1940), pp. 171-72.

[4] Adolf Kaegi, *Life in Ancient India* (Calcutta: Susil Gupta Ltd.), pp. 99-100.

[5] Douglas Guthrie, A *History of Medicine* (Philadelphia: J. B. Lippincott, Co., 1946), p. 92.

dispensary, and a library with six librarians. Fifty speakers recited the Koran day and night without ceasing, while soft music was played to lull the sleepless, and there were storytellers to amuse all. Each patient, upon departure, was given a sum of money, sufficient to tide him over convalescence, until he should be fit to resume work....[6]

Although at this time Europe could boast of great fairs that offered many of the same activities as do county fairs today, and although chivalry was in its heyday, the notion of prevention of dysfunction and the types of treatment cited were not offered in European hospitals. These methods were introduced to the Europeans by Arab physicians of the thirteenth century.[7]

Europe Prior to the Twentieth Century

From Galen's time until the French Revolution, a period of 1500 years, the evidence seems to suggest a constant struggle between the forces opposing man's need for recreation. The literature includes numerous accounts of examples of the decline and rise of a variety of popular recreative activities. At various times a number of laws prohibiting football, golf, dice, cards, and dancing, for example, were enacted; nevertheless, people continued to engage in these activities.

With regard to persons who were ill or disabled, an example of how such prohibitions operated can be found in the Webb's famous report on English Workhouses before 1850:

> There were equally no provision ... for any exercise of mental faculties, either in the form of recreation or in the form of education or training. ... No provision was made for the supply of any books for the use of inmates, whether sick or well, ... no provision was made for playrooms, playthings, or even playing time for children of any age. ... With regard to adults well or sick, it was apparently part of the policy to ignore, and even to prohibit, recreation. Playing cards and all other games of chance were absolutely forbidden to all classes of inmates at all hours and seasons.[8]

This might well be true, but a German national examining these same facilities went back to his country and reported the following:

> In the case of the sick ... not only is the introduction of food and drink forbidden, but also that of books and writings of improper or unsuitable character which may be likely to produce insubordination....

---

[6] Ibid., p. 96.
[7] John L. Lamonte, *The World of the Middle Ages* (New York: Appleton-Century-Crofts, Inc., 1949), p. 561.
[8] Sidney and Beatrice Webb, English Poor Law Policy (London: Longmans, Green and Co. Ltd., 1910), pp. 72-74.
[9] P. F. Aschrott, The English Poor Law System (London: Knight and Co., 1888), pp. 209-11.

> Card playing and games of chance are forbidden; but this prohibition is not very rigidly enforced. In some workhouses, the infirm pass much of their time in playing dominoes and games of the same sort.[9]

The thinking of Philippe Pinel, an eighteenth-century French physician, seems to have had considerable influence on the conscious use of recreative activity for treatment purposes. His theories and treatment regime spread throughout the European continent and through the British Isles, and then to the Western Hemisphere. Pinel and his pupil, Esquirol, taught that with humane treatment and activity, ill persons, and particularly mentally ill persons, would respond and often improve.[10]

Subsequently, a considerable literature regarding recreative activity and mental illness began to appear. W. A. F. Browne, a physician writing in 1837, had this to say about the use of recreative activity:

> It gives regularity to the mental operations, that which nothing can be more conducive to tranquility; it imposes the necessity of self-command and attention, it communicates new series of impressions, and if judiciously managed, it may be made, by giving tone and vigour to the body, to react on the mind in the same manner that evacuants, opiates, or tonics do. It cannot then be immaterial what the nature of the employment is which may be recommended. In the selection, let the object be to combine as many of the objects here specified as possible. It is not enough to have the patients playing the part of busy automatons, or to wear out their muscular energies vicariously, in order to relieve the drooping heart of the load. There must be an active and if possible, intelligent and willing participation on the part of the labourer, and such a portion of interest, amusement, and mental exertion associated with the labour that neither lassitude nor fatigue may follow. The more elevated, the more useful the description of occupation provided then, the better. It ought not to be complicated for that would discourage; it ought not to be purely mechanical, for that frustrates the end in view; it ought not to be useless and evidently for the purpose of acting as a means of abstraction, for the artifice is often detected, and the patient disgusted.[11]

A few years later, a "late inmate of the Glasgow Royal Asylum for Lunatics" published a book which included the following comment regarding recreative activity:

> For the last two years I have attended the concerts and balls given during the dark months of the year to the inmates of Gartnavel Royal Lunatic Asylum; and from what I have seen, and also what I have heard from the inmates themselves, I know that these meetings have often soothed the excited, cheered the desponding, and turned the mind aside for the time from the corroding task of contemplating its own sorrows, and conse-

[10] George W. Albee, *Mental Health Manpower Trends* (New York: Basic Books, Inc., 1959), p. 10.

[11] What Asylums Were, Are, and Ought To Be, *p. 95.*

quently ministered to the great purpose for which asylums are instituted—the cure of insanity.... There are people here listening to the song and joining in the dance—enjoying the clear light, the beauty and fragrance of the fresh evergreens which festoon the hall, who under the old system would have been lying in bonds and darkness—their only music the clanking of the iron bolt and the rattling of the prison keys.[12]

[12] Anonymous, *The Philosophy of Insanity* (Edinburgh: MacLachlan and Stewart, 1860), pp. 65-66.

2
The
Immediate
Past

The Twentieth Century

The notion of recreation as an integral facet of treatment procedures had taken such hold in the treatment of the mentally ill that by 1913 there were numerous published reports of activities for patients, such as the detailed report of a hospital in the United States which chartered a train and took 500 patients on a picnic![1]

During the late nineteenth century, a number of special institutional programs for the mentally retarded were established. At times these were indistinguishable from programs for the mentally ill, but by the turn of the century it was recognized that a variety of recreation techniques could be employed in the "treatment" or "training" of mentally retarded persons. Writing in 1915, the Director of the Vineland, New Jersey institution stated:

> Defectives of all grades lack energy and initiative. They do not therefore, of their own accord, develop the physical coordination that normal children do. Accordingly they must be exercised along these lines if they are to attain to the highest of their limited capacity. Not having the judgement and foresight, the ambition, of normal children, special efforts must be put foward to hold their interest while exercises for coordination are being given. The most natural way to accomplish this is through the medium of games. . . . It should be fully appreciated by teachers, parents, and superintendents that the playing of these games is not "mere play," but *definite training* of the best kind. In many cases there is little else to be done. . . . It should not be forgotten that these games not only develop

[1]*American Journal of Insanity,* 70 (1913), 247-50.

The Immediate Past

coordination and attention, manners, morals, self-control, altruism, patience, and many more desirable qualities are involved.... [These] will help to make him a social rather than an antisocial being![2]

Like the institutions for the mentally ill and the institutions for the mentally retarded, the institutions for the physically ill and disabled offered a variety of recreation services as long as the institutions were kept small and well-endowed.

A number of the special schools for persons who were blind or deaf began to develop recreation services for their students at this time. Formally organized recreation service for persons with visual disability or blindness who were not institutionalized had its genesis in New York City in 1893. One of the founding purposes of the Industrial Home for the Blind was to provide recreation experiences for its clients. Another New York agency—the New York Association for the Blind (commonly known as the Lighthouse)—first began its range of services by providing donated theater and concert tickets for blind adults as early as 1905. The Jewish Guild for the Blind, established in 1914, indicated that one of its original purposes was to provide a recreation center for blind persons.[3]

As each insitution became larger and less able to provide minimum service, recreation service—although vital in certain circumstances—began to wane. This seemed to be the situation in most institutions and particularly the ones under public auspieces.

The advent of war seemed to reverse this process and to affect the growth of recreative experience for institutionalized, as well as noninstitutionalized disabled persons. The military had long recognized the use of recreation as a means of preventing low morale and the resultant ineffective behavior; therefore, it was not surprising that during the Crimean War, Florence Nightingale was able to stimulate the development of recreation service for British troops. She encouraged not only the development of organized recreation service in military camps. but recommended a variety of services for convalescent troops, including the use of pets on a hospital ward.[4]

Consequently, during the First World War, the International Red Cross provided a number of recreation services in military hospitals. By the 1920s the Red Cross organization in the United States employed personnel exclusively for the purpose of providing recreation service in military hospitals, and continues to do this to some degree today.[5]

---

[2] Hilda A. Wrightson, *Games and Exercises for Mental Defectives* (Cambridge, Mass.: Caustic-Chaflin Co., 1916), pp. 1-3.

[3] Maurice Case, *Recreation for Blind Adults* (Springfield, Ill: Charles C. Thomas, Pub., 1966), p. 13.

[4] Florence Nightingale, *Notes on Nursing* (New York: D. Appleton and Company, 1873), pp. 95-104.

[5] Lillian Summers, *The American Red Cross Program of Recreation in Military Hospitals,* Unpublished Master's Thesis, University of North Carolina at Chapel Hill, 1957, 134pp.

Also during this period, an early "text" concerned with recreation and illness was published.[6]

In the early 1930s, a remarkable woman conducted an experiment in the use of recreation in the treatment of the institutionalized mentally retarded. She demonstrated at a large midwestern United States institution for the mentally retarded that an organized program of recreation services can function as a "substitute for former repressive measures of control" and can offer the mentally retarded child an opportunity to develop his ability. Some of her theories, which have been successfully tested, include the following:

1. The course of development of play interests in mentally deficient children is similar to that of normal children up to the level of activities dependent upon the higher intellectual functions, except that the rate of development is slower.
2. The form of play expression is determined somewhat by the environment. In an institutional setting, the game of institution supplants the game of house.
3. There is little correlation between sense of rhythm and ability in motor activities on the one hand, and general intelligence as measured by tests on the other.[7]

The psychoanalytic school of psychology began to have an impact on service in the early 1930s. Titles such as *Emotion and Sport* (1932) and articles such as *Psychoanalytic Theory of Play* (1933) could be found in the literature. A number of theses and dissertations regarding the use of recreative experience in care and treatment of illness and disability also began to appear during this period; for example, *The Selection and Use of Games in Cases of Cardiac Insufficiency* (New York University, 1932).

World War II revitalized recreation service to persons who were ill or disabled. Throughout the world in the late 1940s there were thousands of personnel employed in military and veterans' institutions to provide recreation service. Service was increased to those who were already institutionalized because of blindness, deafness, mental retardation, or mental illness.

> The second World War tragically brought home, to most of the countries in the world, disabled veterans: paraplegics, amputees, and other service disabled casualties.... As part of the vast rehabilitating program, sports were suddenly seen by some as an important aid to rehabilitating the disabled veteran.... In 1948, a few years following the United States' efforts at organizing wheelchair sports, wheelchair athletics took a different path in another country.... Dr. Ludwig Guttman ... at Stoke Manderville, England, saw the value of sports as a therapeutic enhancement. He realized that sports not only aided in the development of unused

---
[6] Neva Boyd, *Hospital and Bedside Games* (Chicago: H. T. Fitzsimmons Co., 1919).
[7] Bertha F. Schlotter, *An Experiment in Recreation with the Mentally Retarded* (Illinois: State Department of Welfare, 1932, revised 1951, reprinted 1956), pp. 142-43.

or atrophied muscles but proved that sports were of immeasurable benefit in maintaining optimum organic fitness and in acquiring functional skills.[8]

Another new service that begun in this period was the development of special community centers that catered to older persons. Although older persons had been involved in organized programs of recreation in multigenerational service agencies for a time, the first Community Center entirely devoted to serving older adults was started by the New York City Department of Welfare in 1944.[9]

In addition, a number of educational institutions in various countries— universities, technical colleges, institutes, and the like—began to organize special programs for those preparing for careers in recreation service to persons who were ill or disabled.

Within the United States a number of other events stimulated practice. In 1953, the University of North Carolina began to host a biannual international seminar on Recreation Services in Hospitals. Under the direction of one of the pioneers in the recreation movement, Professor Harold Meyer, this seminar brought to recreation personnel such notable physicians as Dr. A. R. Martin, former chairman of the American Psychiatric Association Committee on Leisure, and Dr. J. B. Wolffe, former president of the American College of Sports Medicine. Dr. Martin introduced to the recreation field the late Dr. Paul Haun, who through his writings has been a major source of inspiration and influence upon recreation practice in general.

Another equally prominent person who influenced practice in the United States was Beatrice H. Hill, who joined the staff of the National Recreation Association in the early 1950s. Raised in luxury in a philanthropically oriented east coast environment, her education consisted of private schools and tutors. During a period of volunteering in a tuberculosis sanitorium and a personal bout with tuberculosis, her interest was fostered in the development of recreation service for institutionalized persons. She then spent a number of years on New York's Welfare Island at Goldwater Memorial Hospital, as Director of Recreation. She chose to develop ideas in this long-term institution for the chronically ill poor. The results of her experience appears as the now-historic monograph, *Starting a Recreation Program in a Civilian Hospital.* As a consequence she joined the staff of the National Recreation Association, and over a ten-year period built a staff of field consultants who traveled through the United States encouraging the development of recreation services for persons who were ill or disabled. During this time she was instrumental in stimulating the award of public monies for professional education and research in Therapeutic Recreation

---

[8] *The History of Wheelchair Sports* (New York: Joseph Bulova School of Watchmaking, n.d., mimeographed), pp. 1-2.

[9] Susan H. Kubie and Gertrude Landau, *Group Work with the Aged* (New York: International Universities Press, Inc., 1953), p.9.

Service. In 1960, with the advice of her mentor, the noted physiatrist and writer for *The New York Times,* Dr. Howard A. Rusk, she formed a separate national service agency, Comeback, Inc., which expanded the range of her staff's consultation and field service to Canada, Mexico, and various European nations. She was one of the first people to publicly recognize the recreation needs of noninstitutionalized disabled persons, focusing attention on such settings as sheltered workshops, clinics, nursing homes and other residential institutions for the aging, and for others who were homebound or who suffered from alcoholism or drug addiction. Her efforts during this period led to the acceptance of recreation service as a professionally valuable service to those who are ill and disabled.

Simultaneously with these efforts, a number of educational institutions in the United States and Canada established degree and diploma programs for personnel seeking to provide recreation service to disabled persons. Some of these programs specialized in service to aging persons, to persons in correctional institutions, and for service to children.

During the latter half of the sixties, educational programs for recreation personnel began to be concerned with service to disadvantaged persons in urban settings. This development expanded concern for the social dimensions of disability as well as continuing the concern for persons who suffered from disability resulting from disease or trauma.

Recreation service in correctional institutions, although operating for a number of years on a somewhat makeshift basis, began to be expanded in the 1960s.

> Some institutions have developed excellent specialized programs of recreation that have attracted national attention ... the Texas State Penitentiary offers an annual prison rodeo. A prison in Nevada has developed a gambling casino for use by inmates. ... Attendence at outside sporting events is allowed in some institutions. ... Some of the youth institutions have experimented with coed activities, including dances, picnics, movies, and other such activities between boys' and girls' training schools.[10]

In a recent statement regarding services in correctional institutions in the province of Ontario, the following was reported:

> Leisure education is recognized as being of prime importance in assisting those in our care to readjust to life in the community. Recreation programs are therefore being developed to provide a wide variety of physical, social, and cultural activities, with emphasis being placed on the teaching of leisure skills and particularly those activities available in the communities to which the individual will return.[11]

While these events were occurring in the United States and Canada, similar

[10] C. R. Hormachea, "Mission Rehabilitation: The Role of Recreation in the Correctional System," *Therapeutic Recreation Journal,* 3 (1971), 122.

[11] *The Ontario Plan in Corrections,* Ontario Department of Correctional Services, 1970, p. 22.

The Immediate Past

activity occurred in Europe, Austrialia, India, Japan, and elsewhere. For example, a special technical school in Denmark was opened to prepare personnel for recreation service to the mentally retarded and the mentally ill. In Britain, recreation service became reimbursable under the National Health Service. A major general hospital in Stockholm boasted of performances for patients by a symphony orchestra and theater groups, as well as employing a staff member who broadcast special radio programs from the hospital to treatment centers in metropolitan Stockholm.

In South Australia's Parkland hospital, popular musical comedy was staged by patients. Tokyo's Kamasuyama Hospital counts in its program a variety of art and social activities. Mexico City's Hospital Infantil has a rooftop playground and a variety of recreation services.

In Israel, special experimental programs using organized recreation service in the care and treatment of the mentally retarded young adult and the physically impaired adolescent have been initiated.

The Netherlands offers holiday cruises for chronically ill institutionalized persons aboard the special vacation ship the *J. Henry Dunant,* as well as sightseeing tours on a bus fitted with portable respirators for persons who have difficulty breathing. In England, the Spastic Society has developed a program of seaside vacations for clients who are not institutionalized. In Sweden, the Association of the Mentally Retarded hosts a weekend drop-in center for the community. In the United States, a variety of public and private recreation agencies offer special recreation services as well as their general ones to persons with disabilities. In Canada, the agency Recreation for the Handicapped (Montreal) is working on a system for counseling and offering reduced admissions to theaters and sporting events for disabled persons on limited incomes. In the Province of Alberta, a coordinating council has been formed to enable persons with disability to engage in recreative activity in public programs in Edmonton and Calgary.

Many more examples of developments of this type can be cited in the Phillippines, Spain, Finland, and other countries. At the present time, there is probably no place in the world that has not recognized the value of organized recreation service for persons who are ill, institutionalized, disabled, or disadvantaged.

Each nation has developed its own unique system of service delivery, some through the use of elaborate pre-service preparation programs in educational institutions, while others rely mainly on special technical institutes and in-service education. Some make maximum use of recreation as part of their prevention programs, others concentrate on treatment and remedial uses. Some employ specialists in the area of recreation, while others see this as a responsibility of persons in a variety of professions. Regardless of the pattern for delivery of service, each in his own way is interested that service is delivered.

The following chapter examines some of the philosophical contexts in which recreation service is offered to persons who are ill, disabled, or disadvantaged.

3
Principles That Influence Service

Introduction

The phrase *therapeutic recreation service* first appeared in the literature about 1957.[1] It was first coined to distinguish experiences and services offered to persons in special residential settings who were ill, impaired, or had some degree of disability, that prevented them from using recreation resources from services and experiences offered to the public at large in community or neighborhood settings. Later, the phrase referred to services to persons who had special needs, regardless of their place of residence or limitation.

Personnel in therapeutic recreation service were primarily concerned with the situations people found themselves in rather than the resources used for recreation. Service was offered to modify these situations. Emphasis was placed upon the word "service" rather than "recreation" or "therapeutic." The modality for service was usually popular recreative activities including the social norms and behaviors that surrounded these activities. At times, other types of activities were used for "therapeutic" purposes—activities that were supportive of the social situation. Unfortunately, senior administrative personnel in special settings—for example, hospitals, nursing homes, special schools, health departments, and the like—confounded the situation by referring to these efforts as "recreational therapy."

Depending upon the setting and the experience of administrative person-

---

[1] V. Rensvold, B. H. Hill, E. Boggs, M. W. Meyer, "Therapeutic Recreation," *Annals of the Academy of Political and Social Science,* 313 (September 1957), 87-91.

Principles That Influence Service 19

nel, service was seen as a parallel to the many "therapies" offered under the aegis of a physiatrist, such as occupational therapy, physical therapy, corrective therapy, speech therapy, and others. In some settings it was viewed as a type of social work, and more specifically, as transplated social group work. In still other settings, it was identified as adapted physical education, or sometimes as special education. Although there are some common elements in all of these fields, the reality is that they all have vastly different philosophical orientations as well as different types of education and different social missions than do personnel in therapeutic recreation service; nevertheless, confusion between these fields still persists. The following chapter illustrates some of the differences among these fields.

Therapeutic vs. Therapy

Therapeutic recreation service is an area of specialization within the broad field of professional recreation service. Within the context of the recreation field's traditional philosophy, this special area of service modifies traditional approaches and applies knowledge and information from various sciences to enable persons with limitations to engage in recreative experience. Specialists in therapeutic recreation service concern themselves primarily with the human situation rather than limiting concern to activity participation in circumscribed situations. Emphasis is upon the provision of service, framed within the context of the field of recreation and modified to function within various social institutions. Because the *results* of service are nonspecific—theoretically they have a nonspecific effect upon the person rather than a measurable specific effect—they are said to have therapeutic value; however, this effect should not be construed as "therapy" per se. As Haun puts it:

> I like to think of recreation . . . as an important means of increasing the effectiveness of therapy. While not curative in itself, it helps create the milieu for successful treatment. . . . In essence, recreation services help to create in the patient a desirable psychological state by contributing to his self-confidence, his optimism, and his ability to accept the inevitable discomfort of his illness.[2]

In another publication, Haun explains with considerable clarity why "recreation experience" cannot be prescribed in the way that a physician prescribes a therapy for specific treatment purposes:

> The generally understood meaning of a prescription is a written direction for the preparation and use of a medicine . . . to be taken at such and such intervals. A *true* prescription for recreation would have to read something like this:

[2] Haun, *Recreation: a Medical Viewpoint*, pp. 55-56.

Rx John Doe, Ward 18
32 quanta of moderate
pleasure
Sig. 10:00am & 4pm g.d.
for one week.

Richard Roe, M.D.

There are several difficulties in such a prescription. We have no apparatus for the calibration of positive affective states such as pleasure, contentment, and love, or for their opposites. We thus have no reliable concept of a unit of enjoyment or of the varied intensities of wretchedness we are attempting to combat. Neither are we clear as to the distinction, if any, between gladness, cheerfulness, and joy, or whether there are qualitative differences between annoyance, vexation, and irritation.[3]

Unlike other personnel who work with persons suffering from pathology or its residuals, such as nurses, physical therapists, and radiologists, personnel in therapeutic recreation service do not know what the specific result of service will be. It is true that personnel in other professions may make similar statements, because there are individual "patient" reactions; however, generally there are sufficient and accurate data to predict usual finite results from the injection of a drug, the manipulation of a joint, or the administration of radioactive dyes. Recreative experience, on the other hand, is always an individual matter. Service is offered with the understanding that although something may be labeled "recreative," it really may not be recreative for some people. Thus, therapeutic recreation service is generally viewed as a nonspecific treatment with regard to pathology, and is not considered a therapy per se.

Pathology and Its Residuals

When a person is ill, impaired, or disabled, only certain aspects of his personality are limited. He may have a problem with his circulation, for example, or his ambulation may be effected, or his capacity to resist frustration may be decreased. Any number of possible behavioral limitations may be operant as a result of illness, impairment, or disability. Even though this be the case and certain limitations do exist, many aspects of personality still remain intact; that is, they are not effected by illness, impairment, or disability.

Most personnel in health-related professions are primarily concerned with amelioration or modification of behavior with respect to pathology. Personnel in therapeutic recreation service are primarily concerned with nonpathological factors, and therefore focus upon enabling an individual to strengthen aspects of personality that are not affected, in order to prevent further limitation or greater functional loss.

[3] Haun, "Prescribed Recreation," *Recreation in Treatment Centers,* 6, No. 9 (1965), 25-27.

Principles That Influence Service

Further behavioral limitations or greater functional loss is sometimes referred to as "secondary disability." The word "disability" indicates a personal inability to cope with certain aspects of the environment as a result of physical or mental impairment or social barriers. As a consequence of impairment there is loss of function. Impairment may be caused by trauma, defect, disease, or social conditions. Impairment may involve nerve, muscle, bone, or vascular tissue, as well as affect and intellect. When there is absence or death of tissue cells, there is irreversible functional loss. Each impairment is quite specific and differs for every disorder. The residual condition as a result of impairment is permanent and is the primary cause of disability. Permanent sequelae are referred to as *intrinsic residuals.*

However, there are a number of nonspecific sequelae which are not limited to a given disorder and result from neglect, lack of adequate care, and are usually associated with disuse. We are all subject to these sequelae, whether we have a disability or not. Nonspecific sequelae are such phenomena as muscle atrophy, demineralization, circulatory system changes, reflex decrement, decreased bladder and bowel control, periarticular fibrosis, decubitus ulcers, contracture, avitaminosis, and other physical conditions. As a consequence of these conditions there is often decreased cognitive ability and altered affective or emotional response. When someone has been disabled, these nonspecific sequelae complicate the situation and cause further behavioral limitations, which, are often referred to as secondary disability. Secondary disability may be prevented, delayed, limited, or reversed. It is on this premise and with this intent that much of the knowledge and skill of the therapeutic recreation specialist is directed.

Secondary disability need not be a permanent condition, for the residual factors that cause it can be reversed, prevented, or delayed if proper services are made available. When this is not done, there is rapid withdrawal from social interaction and involvement in activities of a social nature. When this happens, one has become handicapped!

The word "handicapped" is supposedly descriptive of a social condition, and in effect expresses our social attitude toward people we so label. The word itself is most intriguing and it is strange how we have come to use it in the English language.

The word "handicap" is a contraction of four English words—*hand in the cap.* The origins of this word are rather obscure, but one dramatic etymological explanation places it prior to the middle of the fourteenth century, and links it with the act of begging.

Through the ages there have always been poor persons who would beg a few coppers from the rich. By the mid-fourteenth century, the number who could not get work in England because of sickness, old age, or a variety of other causes had grown to considerable proportions. Some were truly impaired as a result of work accidents, disease, or military service, while a good many were vagabonds, gypsies, ne'er-do-wells, and able-bodied idlers. It is thought that they begged by standing at the door of a rich person's carriage in a public place and holding forth their caps. A beggar was never sure of what he was given until he put his hand in the cap and pulled out the coins.

We can't be sure of this explanation, but we do know that the problem was so acute that the first of the English Poor Laws, *The Statute of Labours,* was passed in 1350 to help eliminate begging. The famous English epic poem *Piers Plowman,* published a few years later, describes a common gambling game which required the placing of coins in a hat or cap. It calls for no stretch of the imagination to envision people idly playing this game, and when a rich person was seen, stopping the game to beg. We still see laborers at lunch time playing a game which requires pitching pennies into a hat. We still see beggars using their hats as receptacles for money. For our purposes, it is important to note that the origins of "handicap" seem entwined with the notion of gaining something, and that society made no distinction in the cause of begging—a beggar was an undesirable person, regardless of reason.

In the seventeenth century, the word was used as a colloquial expression to indicate financial gain or a similar situation. Here are two poetic examples:

> The Treasurer ... for a price
> Mercates his Maister
>   to extend his purse:
> and handy-capps some Crownes:
> may the boot rise to the boot
>   worthy.
>   (G. DANIEL,
>   *Trinach., Henry V.*
>   xcviii, 1649.)

> Ev'n those who now command,
> The inexorable Roman,
>   were but one step had given:
> Handy-Capps in Fate.
>   (G. DANIEL,
>   *Idyl,* ii, 120, 1653.)

However, the game described in *Piers Plowman* was called *Handycapp* by this time. Samuel Pepys reports this in his *Diary:*

> September 18, 1660,
> To the Miter Taverne in Woodstreete ...
> Here some of us fell to handycapp, a sport that
> I never knew before ...

Did the game come before the begging behavior, or did the begging behavior become institutionalized in the form of a game? It is not uncommon for a social custom to become games. For example, most of us know the game of London Bridge, and have considered it a bit of pleasant nonsense from our childhood. Some anthropologists and folklorists have pointed out, however, that it is neither pleasant nor nonsense. It appears to have been the stylized vestige of the ancient European custom of burying a child alive in the foundation of a new structure, or the offering of a human sacrifice to the gods of the water. The Tug-of-War game that many of us played is thought to be a "degraded miracle play" exemplifying the battle between good and evil. Similarly, some games commemorate courtship methods used by primitive societies, while others are vestiges of many everyday social customs.[4]

Although it seems quite possible that the begging custom was the origin of the game; we have no proof of this.

About the middle of the eighteenth century, the word "handicap" begun to take on a new meaning, as indicated in Pond's *Racing Calendar* of 1754. This publication presented the rules for a horse race called a "Handy-Cap Match":

> A person, holding a hat, suggests that two persons race their horses against one another. The two then put an equal sum in a hat or cap, and then put their hands in their pockets. The person holding the hat specifies the terms of the race. The hands are then taken from their pockets. If they both have nothing in their hands, or both have something in their hands, it is a match. If one has nothing and the other has something, it is not a match ... in any event, the person who suggested the match puts his hand in the cap and draws out all of the money and keeps it.

Obviously this is a direct modification of the game played during the previous century; however, it has one significant difference—the specification of terms. Pond's rules state that "... if a match is made without the weight being mentioned, each horse must carry ten stones. ..." Eventually, the game with the coins and the cap were discarded, and the word was used to refer to the specifications each horse must follow in order to equalize the chances of winning the match.

By 1850, the practice of equalizing chances had spread to many different kinds of games, and included a variety of tactics dealing with weight, space, distance, and the like. In fact, the notion became so generalized that in 1885, the *London Times* stated: "... a high expenditure and heavy taxation handicapps a country."

This usage again seems to suggest a penalty, a disadvantage, a way of specifying an undesirable social situation. Today, the dictionary definition of the word *handicap* indicates that it is

> an artificial disadvantage imposed upon a supposedly superior contestant, or an artificial advantage given to a supposedly inferior contestant

[4] See E. M. Avedon and B. Sutton-Smith, *The Study of Games* (New York: John Wiley & Sons, 1971).

Drawing upon attitudes toward persons who are impaired, and understanding the origin of the word *handicap,* perhaps the definition in relation to disability should read:

> an artificial disadvantage imposed upon a supposedly inferior contestant.

There are many services offered today in relation to intrinsic residuals—services calculated to negate economic inferiority. However, little concern is given to the extrinsic residuals that foster social decrement, particularly service in the area of recreation. Too often when recreation service is provided to persons who are impaired, it is a type of service that focuses on intrinsic residuals and thus reinforces dependency. By gearing such services to the limitations disability imposes, we create artificial disadvantages and prevent the disabled person from utilizing his existing capacities to become a socially independent person. Some people seem to harbor the attitude that the disabled are handicapped—are inferior—and things must be done "for them" and "to them" Perhaps this attitude is operable in some facets of daily life, but it is meaningless in relation to recreation. Thus personnel in therapeutic recreation service focus upon preventing a "handicap" or modifying secondary disability so that it does not "handicap" a person.

Within this context, Campbell sees the provision of therapeutic recreation service on three levels—supportive, re-educative, reconstructive. As a supportive modality, therapeutic recreation service aims to strengthen personality aspects that are not yet affected. As a re-educative modality, focus is upon enabling an individual to make maximal use of existing potentialities even though some limitation is present. As a reconstructive modality, service is tailored to an individual's condition and situation, and is usually a part of an interprofessional effort.

Supportive service is primarily applicable in relation to congenital and chronic physical and mental conditions, in long-term residential settings and community agencies; while re-educative service lends itself to working with persons who are mentally retarded, who must learn to live with altered physical abilities, or who must learn to live in different social structures from those familar to them. Reconstructive service is particularly suited to psychiatric practice and a variety of mental health approaches.[5]

Underlining Principles

A distinguishing characteristic of therapeutic recreation service is that service is based upon the philosophical notion that every man is personally responsible for meeting his own need for recreative experience, regardless of his

---

[5] R. J. Campbell, James Plant, A. R. Martin, and W. Menninger, *Recreation and Psychiatry* (New York: National Recreation Association, 1960), pp. 34-35.

Principles That Influence Service 25

limitations—whether these are exclusively physical, emotional, intellectual, chronological, socioeconomic, or are multidimensional.

Thus it becomes quite clear why one cannot "legislate" recreative experience per se, and why it is impossible to say, "Come to the recreation room and be recreated."

This being the case, it behooves the therapeutic recreation specialist to mobilize his knowledge, abilities, and skills to enable persons to accept the fact that they are responsible for meeting their own needs for recreative experience, if the experience is indeed to be truly recreative. The nature of the experience precludes one person determining this for another. To paraphrase a passage of Eric Fromm's *Man for Himself:*

> A man cannot be recreated by repeating the pattern of other men: he must recreate himself. Man is the only animal that can be bored, that can be discontented, that can feel evicted from paradise. Man is the only animal for whom his own existence is a problem which he has to solve and from which he cannot escape.

Illness, disability, or an impairment does not eliminate this personal responsibility—it complicates it. If this were made clear to children and young persons when they first became limited in some way—and to their families—there would be far fewer adults with overdeveloped recreation dependency needs. All too often one hears complaints from those in residential institutions that there is nothing to do on weekends or in the evenings. Many times persons with disability who reside in the community report that they sit home after they return from the clinic, a workshop, or employment, because they have "nothing to do." Although there are social and architectural and other barriers which inhibit participation and use of community resources for recreation, it becomes evident that many have not been helped to assume their own recreation responsibility, and they are unaware of their own potential for doing something about the recreation problems and the boredom they face.

A second principle which guides the offering of therapeutic recreation service is that every adult requires a personal philosophy of recreation appropriate to his own existential situation. Persons who are limited as a result of physical, psychological, or social factors are often prevented from developing a reality-based personal recreation philosophy because

1. Persons who are limited early in life are usually exposed to situations that reinforce the feeling in themselves and others that there is little they can do. This feeling is further reinforced by circumscribed opportunity for recreative experience and development of recreation skills. As a consequence, they and others underestimate their recreation potential.
2. Persons who become limited during young adulthood and middle life but who previously had extensive recreation experience often encounter experiences during treatment and rehabilitation that are incongru-

ous with their specific socioeconomic and health conditions—conditions that will probably prevail throughout their future lives. As a consequence, they frequently entertain unrealistic views of what they and their families can and should do about recreative needs and what is available to them.
3. Older persons who are psychologically depleted by years of chronic illness, institutionalization, or nonproductive existence in other settings tend to adjust to these conditions by accepting a life of inactivity and boredom. They deal with this by behaving overdependently, apathetically, or by making excessive demands on others rather than involving themselves in meaningful recreative experiences.

To counter these factors, the therapeutic recreation specialist strives to function as a model with respect to social norms, transmitting these norms within a reality-oriented frame of reference and utilizing as many techniques as possible to reinforce social norms. Primary concern is for the current reality situation of the patient or client, and his future reality. For example, if a person has developed a progressive degenerative visual condition that will result in blindness, his recreation experience will undoubtedly be affected, and the specialist would be concerned with the patient's potential ability to cope with the situation. If the situation were one of a temporary nature (as in procedures regarding retinal detachment), emphasis would be placed upon the future and resumption of learned skills and abilities. If the future means permanent visual loss, the patient must become accustomed to a different way of life; he must learn to accept the consequences of this situation, and he must become aware of the set of social attitudes he will face. He must gradually be exposed to the harshness of a society which generally thinks in terms of people who can see. These learnings might initially be accomplished in sheltered situations, later in nonsheltered situations. In contrast, the person who is faced with a temporary problem in lack of vision will be encouraged to use the recovery period in a different way, by building upon the past, planning and exploring areas of recreation involvement in which he has always wanted to engage and now has time for during his period of convalescence.

A similar example would be that of an elderly person in a residential institution who has been placed there against his will and thus steadfastly refuses to become "involved." In this situation, the therapeutic recreation specialist must explicitly recognize the nonvolitional characteristics that are present, and might say, "This is the way you feel, and this is the way it is . . . you can take comfort in misery or can try and find some happiness here!" Any other approach would be dishonest and a disservice. This same principle, seen in an administrative context—in an institution for mentally retarded adults, for example—would discourage any staff effort to structure activity that encourages childlike behavior. In a correctional institution, the principle would preclude programming that was inappropriate with regard to the ethos and socioeconomic frame of reference of the inmates.

It becomes apparent that personnel offering therapeutic recreation service do not function with respect to the primary phenomonological concept of recreation generally operant in the entire field of professional recreation service, but that practice has developed based upon the experiential context of recreation; that is service is not based on the need of people to re-create themselves as a consequence of labor, but rather upon the set of potential effects derived from engaging in various experiences, effects that might influence the behavior of a person because of his current existential situation. Service is usually offered to those persons who are not members of the work force, those who do not "labor," those who have another rationale for "re-creation"—some who did work and others who never will.

Generally, service is not offered in a social institution whose primary responsibility is the provision of opportunities for volitional participation in popular recreative activities. If a person can use these resources, he probably doesn't need the service of a therapeutic recreation specialist. Service is usually offered in settings that have other social functions. Social institutions identified with the field of professional recreation service are primarily viewed as "expressive" institutions in that they offer opportunities for spontaneous, emotionally meaningful, reciprocally empathic experiences. Therapeutic recreation specialists function as "expressive" elements in "instrumental" institutions—institutions that are characterized as being "task-oriented"; for example, hospitals, mental health centers, prisons, homes for the aged, and others.

Service Elements

The specialist in therapeutic recreation service utilizes a number of services in practice. Elements of these services are adapted, modified, and designed to meet the needs of persons with social, physical, and mental limitations with respect to the goal orientations established by the agency under whose auspieces service is offered. These elements may be grouped into four major services:

1. Education and information
2. Stimulation and instruction
3. Resources manipulation
4. Programming and activity leadership

A detailed discussion of these elements of service is presented in Section II.

4
Some Kindred Services

As indicated in Chapter III, in the minds of some administrative personnel there are no differences between therapeutic recreation service and a host of other service fields. This type of blurring often exists among the fields of recreation, education, social work, and the therapies, particularly in an institutional complex that offers service to persons who are ill, impaired, or disabled. Many factors have contributed to this type of thinking—sometimes it has been accidental because of a lack of knowledge, and at other times it is purposive because of budgetary constraints. The primary cause, however, is that all four of these fields make use of popular recreative activity, among other devices, as a vehicle for carrying out their objectives. Although this may be the case, *the use of an activity does not create a profession*—rather it is the rationale for use, including the methods and techniques employed.

It may be fair to say that service professions differ only in their philosophy and their technique. In effect, all use a pool of common knowledge from the social and physical sciences. The rationale or philosophy dictates which knowledges will be taken from the sciences, and it is this "mix" or matrix of knowledges which shapes the field of service. The knowledge and the traditional methods of applying it are what make a profession unique.

The following material attempts to indicate the similarities in these four fields, and to delineate their differences, by examining their goals and objectives, how service is implemented, their clientele, their service settings, and the types of educational preparation they utilize in order to provide service.

I. Recreation

In this context, the word "recreation" refers to an organized network of services calculated to enable individuals to engage in activities that have potential recreative value. This network of services is often grouped into subsets with respect to the specific population groups served or the principal objectives intended for implementation.

FIELD OF SERVICE	OBJECTIVE & GOALS	IMPLEMENTATION	PERSONS SERVED	SETTINGS FOR SERVICE	EDUCATION & PREPARATION
A. Community Recreation Service	offer opportunities for involvement in organized programs generally under public and non-profit auspices	administration, leadership, space, instruction, equipment, facilities, organization	children & adults in multiple & single dwelling units	parks, playgrounds, community centers, schools, "Y," etc.	secondary school, college, university, diploma and degree programs
B. Industrial Recreation Service	offer opportunities for involvement as an employee personnel benefit	same as above and at no cost or minimal charge	employees of industrial corporations	public, private, & commercial resources	preparation in personnel management and related area (might have some preparation in recreation)
C. Church Recreation Service	enhance fellowship and spiritual involvement	organization, space, leadership, some equipment	members of a congregation or parish	churches, synagogues, church related areas	diploma or degree in recreation, theology, religious studies, religious education & others
D. Military Recreation Service	enhance morale and strengthen military organization	similar to Industrial	military personnel and their dependents	public, private, and commercial resources, special facilities or military bases	may have academic preparation in recreation or field of fine & performing arts, or special in-service training

FIELD OF SERVICE	OBJECTIVE & GOALS	IMPLEMENTATION	PERSONS SERVED	SETTINGS FOR SERVICE	EDUCATION & PREPARATION
E. Rural Recreation Service	offer opportunities for organized experience in rural areas	similar to Community	families in agricultural	county office buildings, churches, regional parks, other public rural facilities such as schools	same as Community
F. Commercial Recreation Service	earn profits	entertainment, sale of equipment, skill teaching, rental of facilities, transportation, etc.	anyone with sufficient funds to purchase service	theaters, concert halls, arenas, resorts, bowling alleys, stadia, amusement parks, pubs, circuses, taverns, rodeos restaurants, etc.	nonspecific, may have academic preparation or training in art, music, sports, travel, business, hotel management, etc.
G. Outdoor Recreation Service	offer opportunities for experience in a natural environment	same as Community	children & adults	woodland areas, lakes, streams, campsites, snow areas, trails, mountains, seashore, etc.	same as Community with special concentration
H. Therapeutic Recreation Service	promote health, prevent secondary disability, modify or ameliorate illness and disadvantage	administration, leadership, instruction, counseling, consultation facility modification, activity & equipment adaptation	children & adults who are ill, impaired, disabled, disadvantaged because of physical, mental, or social pathology	residential institutions, hospitals, nursing homes, special schools for the retarded & the blind, correctional institutions, homes for the aging, senior centers, rehabilitation institutions, & the like	same as Community with special concentration

II. Education

Education is the process by which an individual develops and cultivates the information, knowledge, and skill that his society believes necessary for individual and collective survival. The word "education" is used more often in English-speaking countries to indicate the formal process of disciplining the mind through systematic instruction and teaching, a process more appropriately called "schooling." Apart from schooling, all aspects of culture educate an individual, particularly the mass media, travel, child-rearing practices, and many other things. Some fields of education are more closely linked to recreation service in that the information, knowledge, and skill that an individual develops or cultivates through the process of schooling can be used by participants in popular recreative activities. The following, although not an exhaustive list of education fields, seem to be closely related to the field of recreation service in the thinking of the average citizen.

FIELD OF SERVICE	OBJECTIVES & GOALS	IMPLEMENTATION	PERSONS SERVED	SETTINGS FOR SERVICE	EDUCATION & PREPARATION
A. Informal, Community, After-school, Leisure Education; Intramural, Intermural, Extramural, Co-Curriculum, Extracurricular Activity	to teach subject matter having implications for recreative involvement in adult life; to provide opportunity to learn and practice skills relating to popular recreative activity	administration, organization, teaching-learning process, guidance, equipment, supplies facilities, financing	average primary, secondary, undergraduate students	schools and school-owned facilities	university and/or teacher training programs
B. Adult Education	to offer opportunity for continuous educational experience, primarily of a non-vocational content	administration, organization, teaching-learning process, lectures, discussions, readings, etc.	average adults who have completed formal schooling	schools, community centers, churches, etc.	nonspecific
C. Special Education	to offer formal instructional opportunities to persons who are exceptional or disadvantaged	adapted teaching-learning technique, and other modified educational methods and procedures	children & youth who are physically disabled, emotionally disturbed, mentally retarded, socially limited, or intellectually gifted	schools and residential	university and/or teacher training

FIELD OF SERVICE	OBJECTIVES & GOALS	IMPLEMENTATION	PERSONS SERVED	SETTINGS FOR SERVICE	EDUCATION & PREPARATION
D. Outdoor Education	to offer opportunity for educational experiences outside the classroom using the natural environment as part of the subject matter to be taught; to develop an appreciation of the natural environment	adapted teaching-learning process, camping	children and teenagers	campsites, woodland areas, regional and national parks, school ships, etc.	university
E. Physical Education	to teach people about the physical use of self in exercise, conditioning, athletics, sports, and how to develop skill in these areas	teaching-learning process	average children, teenagers, and young adults	public schools and other educational settings such as boarding schools, colleges, etc.	teacher training
F. Adaptive Physical Education	to offer exceptional individuals an opportunity for physical education	adapted teaching-learning process	children and teenagers who are disabled or impaired	public schools and residential settings for exceptional persons	teacher training
G. Corrective Physical Education	to treat physical disability	exercise and conditioning	children and adults	clinics, schools, hospitals, etc.	teacher training and special educational preparation

Some Kindred Services 35

Other educational fields concerned with specific content related to recreation include such fields as music, art, dance, drama, home and family life, religion, and others.

III. Social Work

The application of specific information from the social sciences to assist individuals and groups to meet individual and communal needs through a process designated as "the helping process" delineates the profession of social work. Procedures are classified as case work when service is given to an individual, group work when service is offered to an aggregrate of individuals, sometimes as clinical social work when offered in a medical setting, and sometimes as intergroup work when concerned with multi-ethnic groups. Because some recreative experiences are of an intragroup nature and often administered in private agencies and other community resources that employ personnel who are trained in the practice of social work, this practice is related to the field of recreation.

FIELD OF SERVICE	OBJECTIVE & GOALS	IMPLEMENTATION	PERSONS SERVED	SETTINGS FOR SERVICE	EDUCATION & PREPARATION
A. Social Group Work	to direct the interaction between members of a group toward accomplishment of predetermined goals and objectives of the group sponsor	the helping process	average children and adults	private and non-agencies; i.e., Sunday-School class, hospital nursing team, industrial production group, boys' stamp-collecting club, outpatient psychotherapy group, and the like	university
B. Community Organization and Administration	to facilitate the organization and administration of service by use of social work methods	the helping process	professional staff members of local and regional agencies	social work agencies	university

Some Kindred Services

IV. Treatment Services

Care and treatment services use a variety of media in the course of helping to improve the health of a patient. Some of these media are also used by other fields of service and other professions. *The use of the media in itself does not distinguish these services, nor does it create a profession.* Rather, it is the objectives for use of the media and the methods of use which create a profession. Some care and treatment services often use media that may result in a recreative experience, or that may be popularly thought of as "recreation"— thus some of these services are related to the field of recreation.

FIELD OF SERVICE	OBJECTIVE & GOALS	IMPLEMENTATION	PERSONS SERVED	SETTINGS FOR SERVICE	EDUCATION & PREPARATION
A. Physical Therapy	to treat specific musculo-skeletal disorders under a physician's prescription	heat, cold, light, manipulation, exercise, massage	anyone for whom a physician prescribes such service	hospitals, clinics, nursing homes, etc.	technical education or university
B. Occupational Therapy	to treat specific musculo-skeletal disorders, mental illness, and conduct prevocational evaluations and teach activities of daily living under the direction of a physician	utilization of kinetic aspects of a range of occupational pursuits	same as physical therapy		
C. Corrective Therapy	to assist in the treatment of musculo-skeletal disorders	exercise, conditioning drills, athletics	same as physical therapy		
D. Play Therapy	to permit non-verbal expression of emotional conflict	games, dolls, household items, toys, etc.	young children	office, out-patient clinic, or hospital	psychologist, psychiatrist, social worker, or nurse
E. Music Therapy Dance Therapy Drama Therapy Art Therapy	to treat mental illness through the use of a specific experience and interpretation	each service uses the activity itself	usually adults	psychiatric hospitals	nonspecific

F. Activity Therapy: collective term used in many psychiatric settings to group all of the above therapies (A-E) for administrative purposes.

Some Kindred Services 39

The following section examines elements of therapeutic recreation service in detail, and offers information from the social and behavioral sciences which forms the knowledge and skill base for service.

II
THE KNOWLEDGE AND SKILL BASE FOR SERVICE

All service fields, from law enforcement to hotel management, have a body of knowledge and a range of techniques for providing service. The extent of knowledge and technique depends upon the intensity of service provided to the public, the amount of available information about the particular service, and the age of the service field. For example, how complex is the provision of service, how much scientific fact and theory has been made available in the specific area of concern, and how many traditions have grown up around the practice itself?

Relatively speaking, the practice of therapeutic recreation service can be quite complex, dependent upon a host of factors. As service becomes more complex, a larger body of knowledge and theory must be utilized. However, although the roots of practice are in ancient history, current practice is relatively young and is not hampered by obsolete traditions and service models. Furthermore, because recreation per se has a strong relationship to culture, there is still considerable variation from society to society.

This section identifies the elements of therapeutic recreation service and indicates the general and specific tasks that recreation specialist are asked to perform. Some of these tasks are general and nonspecific with respect to a setting, be it a hospital, school, correctional institution, or community agency. Other tasks are quite specific with regard to setting. Certain tasks are general and nonspecific with respect to the service recipient—children, adults, elderly person, men, women, persons with physical disability, the mentally ill, the mentally retarded, the institutionalized, persons in correctional settings, and others. In contrast, certain tasks are specific with respect to a given life situation or condition.

Subsequent chapters of Section II include information regarding the knowledges drawn from the sciences that form the bases for the provision of therapeutic recreation service and provide an enumeration of the application of these knowledges to practice.

5
Aspects of Recreation

In attempting to determine knowledges and skills necessary for the practice of therapeutic recreation service, it becomes apparent that a sharp delineation of the characteristics of recreation must first be made. From a linguistic point of view, the word "recreation" is used in four different ways or contexts:

I. Philosophical
II. Experience
III. Social Institution
IV. Service

Recreation as a Philosophical Concept

Some people use the word "recreation" as the name of an idea, a theory, or a philosophical concept. This notion has been described and continues to be described in semantic terms with attempts at universal definition, consumes an infinite number of pages in the literature, and thrives on endless hours of debate at meetings and conferences, in the classroom, and in the conversations and thoughts of people in all walks of life.

What is the relationship of this philosophical construct to other concepts, such as leisure and hedonism?

What are the historical antecedents of this concept, and how has the concept evolved?

Is this a static or dynamic concept? Is it viable in contemporary society?

How does this concept relate to the practice of therapeutic recreation service?

Generally, the notion of a need to "re-create" oneself has its roots and sanction in the Protestant Reformation. The notion was apparently born when value was placed upon labor and employment that contributed to the economic structure of life in preference to earlier valued notions such as leisure, contemplation, meditation, and other self-indulgent behaviors. Thus, English language dictionaries tell us that "recreation" means "refreshment of mind and body after toil and labor." The followers of Luther and Calvin further qualified this notion by implying that recreation was a reward for labor and toil well done.[1]

Recreation implied activity that was not related to man's central collective obligatory tasks, but rather activity that was voluntarily chosen and self-indulgent, activity that was restorative and offered a degree of enjoyment or release from the burdens of responsibility. Leisure in a classical sense implied a way of living, a state of being in which one had time to contemplate his relationship to God without having to be concerned with obligations and responsibility. This was a state few people had or could ever hope to attain. The Protestant Reformation affirmed that labor and toil was the *primary* way to salvation, and thus the "leisure state" became the time when every man could engage in such a behavior as recreation. With this reversal in values, such notions as hedonism—the pursuit of pleasure either on a sensual or cognitive plane, or the pursuit of a painless existence—became negative, and "playing" was considered a waste of important time. Contemplation was idleness, and encouraged satanically inspired behavior. Recreation then took on a very "active" form, a form which resembled the values of labor and toil per se.

In contemporary society, there is apparently a lessening of emphasis upon obligatory labor and toil as the central focus of every man's existence, but there still seems to be somewhat of an overlay of this form in popular thinking about recreation—thinking that has created an almost frenetic involvement in activity. Idleness and contemplation still appear to have little value and thus all men—well or ill, able or disabled—are encouraged to develop an active recreation pattern.[2]

As toil and labor become less routine and less time is spent in obligatory tasks, contemplation and idleness may once again be valued. However, because technology seems to be fostering an increase in maintenance time, this may not

---

[1] See Adriano Tilgher, *Homo Farber—Work: What It Has Meant to Men throughout the Ages* (London: George P. Harras and Co., Ltd., 1931); and Max Weber, *The Protestant Ethic and the Spirit of Capitalism* (London: G. Allen and Unwin, Ltd., 1930); see also G.J. Dahl, "Time, Work, and Leisure Today," *The Christian Century,* 88(6), 2/10/71, p. 185-89.

[2] For a more detailed discussion of this aspect, see Richard G. Kraus, *Leisure and Recreation in Modern Society* (New York: Appleton-Century-Crofts, 1971), pp. 260-63.

Recreation as an Experience

To the average person—child, young adult, mature adult, older adult—*recreation* is a label placed on a subjective psychological experience that manifests itself while one is engaging in a variety of activities.

What is the nature of this experience? What stimulates it? What deters it? How does it respond and function with respect to a given existential situation? How is the experience manifested in behavioral phenomena? What is the effect of pathology upon the experience? What is the effect of the experience upon pathology? What are the implications of these experiences with respect to bio-psycho-social development and functioning of the individual?

Felix M. Kessing, an anthropologist, described the behavioral zone that most people label "recreation" in this manner:

> It is strongly marked by fictional premises, by elective variation, by risktaking, by the super-utilitarian, by the non-serious, by relative freedom from demanding goal-orientation and strong sanction. It is far-ranging, with many possible types of structured group activity, yet also much that is informal and personal, as with humor, fantasy, or even "just sitting around." Like magic it has what might be called "white" facets of public, approved behavior, and also "black" facets of private, subversive behavior as with salacity, pornography, and obscenity. . . .
>
> In terms of function, a particular kind of recreation may activate in varing degree such elements as (1) pleasurable or hedonistic affects, which are likely to be stressed; (2) organically relaxing, energy-restoring results in the busy or tired person, or an outlet for excess energy in the case of the zestful; (3) integrative or reinforcing influences upon individual or group making for stability or cohesion, or high morale; (4) therapeutic or sublimative results as often channeling off conflict, aggression, or hostilities; (5) creative or reintegrative tendencies, as offering fields for nimble innovation and self-expression; (6) communicative functions, as in learning and habit formation, notable among children, but also among adults; and (7) a frequently symbolic significance, as in playing out important cultural values and premises, e.g., as with many toys.[5]

Anything and everything offers opportunities for recreative experience.

---

[3] See Stefan Lindner, *The Harried Leisure Class* (New York: Columbia University Press, 1970).

[4] See Stanley Parker, *The Future of Work and Leisure* (London: MacGibbon and Kee, 1971).

[5] "Recreative Behavior and Culture Change," *Men and Cultures*, A. F. Wallace, ed., Papers of the 5th Congress of Anthropological and Ethnological Sciences, 1956 (Philadelphia: University of Pennsylvania Press, 1960), p. 131.

Civilization has retained some activities for the sheer joy they bring. Activities that serve no physical survival purpose other than recreation are called "recreation activities," such as games and sports.

However, as many of us have found, a number of activities that can have a survival or utilitarian purpose in civilization can also have recreative value for certain individuals—for example, cooking, sewing, and building. This is indeed so because recreation per se is a psychic phenomenon, subject only to our own psychic organization of experience. Value is the result of how we feel about an activity, or how we perceive a task to be performed. All activity is really neutral in that the values we ascribe to it are the consequences of our own thinking and past experience. Thus "recreation" per se is an internal, psychic phenomenon, and is a different, individualized experience for each of us. That which we collectively label "recreation" is the result of a social convention, and is really only an approximation, because the experience is different for each of us.

As a psychic experience, recreation may be characterized by irrationality, intuitive insight, a sense of authority, affirmation, transcendence, impersonal tone, exaltation, momentariness, and immediacy.

1. Recreation is irrational in that it defies reasoning and intellect. A person cannot explain why an experience is recreative one day and not the next, or what makes a certain situation recreative for him.
2. Recreation generates intuitive insight in that it evokes a new kind of cognition of one's self, a seeing of one's self in another perspective.
3. Because recreation is so direct and personal, it gives one a sense of authority. When one has this sense of authority, an experience is affirmative in one's own eyes.
4. In recreative experience, the everyday, the routine, and the mundane are transcended. A person does not feel that only he can have this experience. On the contrary, he wishes to share it, and wants others to partake of it. Although the phenomenon is personal, it is characterized by an impersonal tone because the participant feels it can happen to anyone.
5. In a recreative experience a person may be raised to a state of exaltation, freedom, and feelings of fulfillment. Through the experience a person's ordinarily limited reality orientation alters, and he becomes part of the larger reality.
6. The essence of recreation is abrupt and momentary. It happens and is gone. One tries to recapture it, but cannot, and then abruptly it comes again.
7. Recreation is characterized by immediacy, for it is directly and consciously present. When it exists, the person is consciously aware that he is involved in it and is a part of it, and that it is happening to him.

Recreative experience does not appear to restrict itself as to time, place, or act, but it does require that the person be both subject and agent of the experience, or affirmer and affirmed of the act.

1. The phenomenon may occur at any time—day or night, in any place, position, location, during any act—while playing, working, resting, traveling, eating, being entertained, loving.
2. To experience recreation, one must engage in some act—one must be the moving force as well as the instrument of the phenomenon. To be the subject of the experience, one must be the agent who enters into and controls the experience.

Thus, recreation is generated from within oneself, interacts within oneself, and remains within oneself. Another person may act as a catalyst, a specific object or act may have an attracting valence quality, but no force outside of the self can make a person experience recreation.

Recreation as a Social Institution

Others identify recreation as collective behavior within specific social structures. These people consider recreation a social institution, and they indicate that as in the case of other social institutions. recreation has form, structure, traditions, patterns of operation and association, systems of communication, and a number of other fixed societal aspects. Some scholars feel that recreation is not a social institution in its own right—does not have a fixed form—but rather attaches itself to other institutions in society.

In an institutional sense, what are the social functions of recreation?

What are its structural and organizational components; how does it articulate with other social institutions?

What variations and modifications in structure exist with regard to ecological, national, ethnic, economic, and other social variables?

What are the sociopathic implications of this institution?

What degree of social control does this institution exert in contemporary society?

From a sociological perspective, principally within the United States, Canada, England, Sweden, Japan, and to a lesser extent in Continental Europe, recreation may be viewed within the context of formal organization theory. A cadre of personnel utilizing many different and diverse knowledges and skills are employed to enable the public to experience recreation. Often referred to as the "recreation movement," this organization of personnel is historically unusual and unprecedented, in that a similar organizational structure of such magnitude has never existed in society prior to this century. The business of providing opportunities for recreative experience in the past has for the most part been one of the functions of the family, the home, and later on, in cooperation with one's immediate neighbors, and then with one's parish and fellow members of a religious congregation. Today, recreation opportunities are provided to "strangers" by "strangers" in an organized system of services which takes on the dimensions of a social institution.

A social institution in a sociological context is a vital interest or activity surrounded by a cluster of mores and folkways, such as marriage and childrearing. A social institution is a formal relationship pattern sanctioned by society, a form and structure that arises and persists because of a definite felt need of the members of society, as in the case of education and schooling. This structure embodies the means or modus operandi for the control of social energy in that it is a deliberately accepted method of attaining a deliberately approved end, as in the realm of health and the creation of a medical and hospital system. A social institution is not just a concept or an idea as such, or a social interest, for that matter; it is a formal structure and apparatus that includes social functionaries (personnel) who through the structure attempt to serve the needs of society.

No social institution arises unless society recognizes the need for it, and although society no longer has certain needs, some social institutions continue to exist and are mere relics of the past. Some institutions concern themselves with esthetic and expressive needs of society, for example, while others concern themselves with communicative, ethical, and economic needs of society. Recreation embodies a structure and function that seeks to meet the recreative needs of society; however, some sociologists maintain that recreation is not yet a social institution because it does not possess the degree of "fixity" present in most established social institutions. To some minds, this is a positive state of affairs. Dr. James Plant, a psychiatrist writing in the 1930s, indicated:

> You can develop the rhythms of persons or you can follow the path of history toward disintegrating people through imposing rhythms upon them.... You do not stand at a crossroads, your choice here is not one just for 1937 ... this is a struggle of the next ten and twenty and thirty years.... To build ever more magnificent programs of recreation ... will bring you rewards in the coin of the realm ... but it will be selling your birthright for a mess of pottage.[6]

Nor was the issue of fixity an issue only in Plant's time; more than twenty years later, in a similar paper, another psychiatrist, Dr. A. R. Martin, commented:

> Unless the recreator has a positive health promotion conception of leisure and recreation, recreation will operate solely on ... a kind of L.P.A.—Leisure Projects Administration—to provide occupations for the spiritually unemployed ... primarily to be functionaries in L.P.A. projects....[7]

What appears to be the mission of the functionaries in the recreation

---

[6] "Recreation and the Social Integration of the Individual," *Recreation and Psychiatry* (New York: National Recreation Association, 1960), p. 7.

[7] "Recreation a Positive Force in Preventive Medicine", *Recreation and Psychiatry* (New York: National Recreation Association, 1960), p. 31.

Aspects of Recreation

movement? What specifically are the social functions of recreation? What social needs does recreation in an institutional context seek to meet?

Kessing has suggested seven major functions (see p. 45), while Roberts, a sociologist, suggests that the function of recreation is primarily to offer a means of social control. It allows the expression of feelings and the release of tension through a range of activity which allows for individual differences. At the same time, recreation exposes people to a value system that upholds the social order.[8]

On the other hand, Richard Kraus, a prolific spokesman for the professional recreation personnel in the United States, indicates a broad range of social functions with respect to contemporary social issues; namely

Improving
    the total quality of community life
    the quality of the environment
    intergroup relations

Contributing to
    the economy
    mental health
    physical health
    special needs of subgroups in society; e.g., the mentally retarded, the disabled, the aging, the delinquent

Providing
    social opportunities
    an outlet for violence
    alternatives to socially harmful activities

Kraus also indicates that in addition to these functions, organized recreation has a responsibility to meet the need for public ritual.[9]

Apparently, each authority has a view of recreation's social function within his own frame of reference; however, it is clear that recreation in a social institutional context attempts to respond to a number of recognized social needs, and thus its form and structure are molded and service is influenced by the social needs that are responded to!

Structurally, recreation can be differentiated from other social institutions. Local, regional, and national authorities provide such loci of concern as parks, community centers, museums, libraries, zoos, aquaria, stadia, arenas, pools, beaches, and a host of other resources. Private groups band together in such structurers as the "Y," Scouts, country clubs, and other special-interest groups. Commercial groups devise many structures running the gamut from the motion-picture industry to retail outlets for the sale of hobby and sport supplies.

[8] Kenneth Roberts, *Leisure* (London: Longman Group Ltd., 1970), Chapter 8.
[9] Richard G. Kraus, *Recreation and Leisure in Modern Society*, Chapter 17.

Professional groups, unions, and a variety of membership organizations responsible for attempting to meet social needs for recreation exercise their own influence upon the manner in which the need is met. A form and structure is established which attempts to satisfy public demand, but because public taste and fancy is somewhat unpredictable, a fixed form and structure is somewhat detrimental to the groups concerned. Thus an intricate network of journals, meetings, conferences, newsletters, and other communication devices have developed to keep personnel abreast of trends and influences.

It has been suggested that because of the variability in public taste, recreation should attempt to standardize public interest in order to serve the widest possible markets. There is, as a consequence, a neglect of minority taste and a striving to find a common denominator. Governments on the one hand encourage and discourage certain aspects of recreation, pandering to some and rejecting others, while private groups dominated by economic forces tend to a great extent to encourage conformity.

In addition to social structures and organizations whose primary role and function in society is to meet needs for recreation, there are other social institutions that have different primary roles but nevertheless attempt to meet the need for recreation. These are such institutions as schools, hospitals, correctional institutions, and the like. These institutions, although meeting a social need for recreation, view this secondary responsibility in terms of their primary social responsibility, and therefore treat recreation as a means to another objective rather than as an end in itself. In the past, there has been minimal articulation between the so-called "recreation agencies" and agencies providing recreation service, but this picture has been changing somewhat, particularly with the advent of formal pre-service educational programs.

With respect to ecological factors, variation in structure is pronounced, but less so than early in the development of the recreation movement. More formally differentiated institutions exist in urban settings, while less formally differentiated institutions exist in rural areas. For example, most municipalities have public recreation departments, while a rural county or region might attempt to meet recreation needs through a school district, an agricultural extention program, a health department, or a farm cooperative. National variations seem to parallel industrial and economic development. Those nations considered "post-industrial" appear to have sharply differentiated recreation institutions, while the "pre-industrial" ones do not. Ethnic factors seemed to have played a large part in the organization of recreation institutions in the past, but less so today. In fact, the dominant social factor appears to be economic. There is universal recognition of the need for opportunities for recreative experience, but economic forces seem to govern to a great extent how this need will be met.

Interest groups cannot generally support the structure for meeting their own need for recreation. For example, football players can not personally afford to maintain the physical space required for playing any more than concertgoers can support a symphony orchestra. Thus governments must supplement and

Aspects of Recreation

augment any structure calculated to meet recreation needs today. This results in patronage at the expense of the remainder of society, and such issues as whether to build a new opera house or maintain more open space for a golf course result in sharp debate in legislative assemblies.

Earlier in this century, texts concerned with the provision of organized recreation stressed its functional relationship to the "worthy use of leisure." It was felt by some that drinking, gambling, dancing, and other leisure activities of this ilk were not a proper use of one's time. Organized recreation was on "the side of the angels." Thus, professional recreation personnel in the public and nonprofit sphere have been closely identified with "character building," while their colleagues in the commercial recreation field have been somewhat looked down upon. Pool halls and billiard pallors, bowling alleys and dance halls were once considered unsavory places which nice people didn't frequent. Today, all of these places are acceptable resources for recreation. Very few resources which the recreation movement offers the public today can be considered sociopathic. On the contrary, regardless of auspices, public or proprietary, private or commercial organized recreation in itself is well thought of and supported by society. However, there are those who feel that the opportunity and provision for too much recreation tends to morally weaken society—thus they speak of recreation as a means for "curing" social ills; i.e., keeping people "fit," keeping the would-be delinquent off the street, helping the laborer to recapitulate. Some feel that because of the need to provide for so many people with such a diversity of interests, the minimal resources at hand limit the quality of the experiences, and ultimately cultural values are undermined. Excellence in esthetics are sacrificed at the expense of allowing as many people as possible to "get involved."

Finally, there are those who find in some socially acceptable recreation pursuits opportunities for the reinforcement of psychopathology; they label such experiences as destructive to society. This factor runs the course from the destruction of the environment to the destruction of self under the guise of recreation.

Recreation as a Service

Because recreation is offered to the public through a structured network of services, some identify these specific services as "recreation services." Some of these services require a high degree of preparation and proficiency for effective practice, while others require limited knowledge and ability. Many recreation services are primarily educative, while some are essentially manipulative and administrative.

What is the nature of a given service; how does each service relate to the others; what is the interrelationship of service?

What modifications must a given service undergo in order to be operable in a particular institutional setting?

What is the effect of a given service in relation to a given objective?

What are the required elements of educational preparation in order to offer adequate and effective service?

How does the communication process affect the provision of service?

What influence do such variables as technology, life style, taste, mores, and others have upon the utilization of specific services?

What are the therapeutic implications of specific services?

Primary recreation service elements are (1) administrative, (2) supervisory, (3) leadership, (4) consultative, (5) coordinative, and (6) research.

Administrative services are primarily concerned with the efficient execution of agency policy and program implementation. As a consequence, administrative tasks focus upon budgetary and personnel considerations that are basic to program effectiveness. Supervisory services imply a knowledge of the parameters of effective personnel performance and the setting of expectations with respect to patient and client services. Leadership services concern the direct interaction of personnel with patients and clients regarding specific program goals. Consultative services provide for the interaction of two professional persons to enhance direct service to patients or clients. Coordinative services imply a degree of collaboration between two or more professional persons who are engaged in the provision of direct service to patients or clients. Research services find application either in the process of total service delivery or in evaluation of patient or client need, participant response to service, or program effectiveness.

Service modifications occur with respect to the primary "mission" of a given institution in which service is offered. For example, when therapeutic recreation service is offered in an educational institution, basic concerns are with education; in a health institution, the concern is with health. In long-term care settings, the concern centers around the total living situation of particular patients or clients. Although service may be designed with specific clinical goals for a given patient or client, these are offered within the "mission orientation" of the host institution. Subsequent chapters present material regarding these modifications.

All services must be offered with a goal orientation regardless of the type of institution in which they are offered. Patients or clients who use a given "task-oriented" institution do so for specific reasons—none of which are for recreative experience. It behooves the therapeutic recreation specialist to design his services so that they are calculated to contribute to this goal orientation.

Supportive services can be effectively offered by a variety of personnel with little special educational preparation for this task, provided they are under good supervision. Indeed, personnel from a variety of fields contribute to supportive services. Re-educative services require a degree of formal preparation that includes some knowledge of the pathological processes of concern and an ability to communicate with other professional members of the staff. Reconstructive services require a high degree of professional preparation and a

Aspects of Recreation

considerable knowledge of how pathology influences behavior. Specific educational programs designed to prepare personnel for these levels of service vary, dependant upon the educational system for preparation operant in a given nation. In the United States and Canada, for example, educational preparation for therapeutic recreation service is conducted in community colleges and universities. In Denmark and the Netherlands it is offered in special technical institutes.

Because the condition of a patient or client is dynamic, considerable communication must be part of an ongoing process within any structure. Recreation personnel cannot work in a professional vacuum and must consistently communicate with other professional persons serving the same clients and patients. In turn, these other personnel must consistently communicate with recreation personnel. Lack of communication tends to impede the therapeutic process.

A number of social variables such as technology, life style, and so forth will exert considerable influence upon the provision of service. For example, using advanced methods of communicating findings or reporting progress will lessen paperwork and increase time spent in direct service. Factors such as life style will exert influence on the nature of the total recreation program. If patient or client life style is different from staff life style, this will affect rapport, participation, and a number of other factors. Mores of a given institution will exert influence upon specific services. Subsequent chapters will discuss these factors in more detail.

The following chapters in this section amplify some of the material contained in this chapter. Chapters VI and VII present a detailed examination of the elements of therapeutic recreation service, indicating which tasks are nonspecific with respect to setting or person and which tasks are specific with regard to setting and/or care and treatment goals. Subsequent chapters are concerned with specific aspects of the sciences that form the knowledge base used in practice.

6
Elements of Service
Part I

There are four major elements of service: education and information, stimulation and instruction, manipulation of resources, and programming and the conduct of activity. These four groups embody a number of tasks which personnel perform. Some of these tasks are nonspecific with regard to the presenting situation of the service recipient and are generally applicable in all settings. However, some tasks are quite specific, and vary with respect to the setting, care pattern, and treatment goals.

Education and Information

Based on the principle of *personal responsibility for meeting one's own need for recreative experience,* the specialist in therapeutic recreation service offers *education to develop awareness of personal responsibility.* A range of techniques may be employed in this undertaking, from general discussion on a one-to-one basis with the patient or client to a series of experiences calculated to generate insight regarding personal responsibility. For example:

"Is this the Recreation Department?" asked a rather portly gentleman in pajamas and robe, as he came into the office.

"Yes, can I help you?" I said, putting down my pen and looking up from my desk. "Won't you sit down?"

The man sat and introduced himself. He was a patient on Ward 16, and one of the nurses had suggested that he come down and talk with me. "I've been here three weeks now, and they say I might be here another three," he mumbled with an edge in his voice. "I need something to do, they only give me treatments in the morning, and I have all afternoon and evening to myself. On the weekends, it's worse. I'm tired of reading the newspapers. I want something to do!"

"What would you like to do?" I asked.

"You tell me," he retorted angrily, "you're the recreation expert."

"Well, there are a number of regular activities which we schedule each week. Here," I said with wonder, handing him the printed weekly schedule, "haven't you been given one of these?"

"Yes, they deliver one each week, but there's very little on the list that interests me, and besides, no one has invited me to come to these events, who's supposed to do that?"

"No one—the activities listed are open to any patient who wants to come to them whose physician has given permission for him to attend. Didn't the nurse tell you that?"

"I suppose so, something like that, but I'm not interested in discussion groups, or making things, or playing cards, and things like that. I'd rather watch TV."

"Well, why don't you?"

"I get bored. I've been watching it almost all day, every day, except when I read the papers, or nap, or when they take me for treatments. There must be something more entertaining to do—this *is* the Recreation Department!"

"Yes, this is the Recreation Department, but we're not miracle workers. We schedule a number of activities each week which have general interest. In fact, it is a rather extensive list by a number of standards. However, it is possible that you may not find anything on the schedule that interests you. What do you think you would like to do? Maybe we can help you get started. There may be other patients in the hospital at this time who have expressed similar interests."

"I don't know—I don't do much at home. When I get home from work, I watch TV after supper, while my wife does the dishes, then she joins me and we watch until the late news is over, and then we go to bed."

"Do you do this every day, and nothing else?"

"Oh, we used to go to the movies, but it's too much of a hassle, and besides, the TV has the same things. Once in a while, we take a walk, if the weather is warm, and of course in the summer we do go to the beach sometimes."

"Is that all? No friends, no parties, no relatives?"

"Well, we do get together with some friends once in a while, but then we sit around and have a beer and talk or watch TV. I used to play a little poker, but I don't find that very interesting any more. In fact, if my wife didn't make arrangements, we'd never do anything, I suppose."

"Your wife is your recreation director, you might say."

"Well, you could say that, I suppose. What are you getting at?"

"It seems to me that while you are here in the hospital, you'll have to be your own recreation director. You have a list of activities, and you'll have to make use of it yourself, if you want to do anything. If you don't want to do what is on the list, then you can request something else you would like to do, and we will try to oblige. But you will have to do the scheduling and requesting for yourself. No one here is going to do that for you."

In this example, the specialist used a direct approach to bring to the patient's attention his current recreation pattern and his responsibility in maintaining it if he wanted to. He indicated that the patient's discomfort would remain unless he (the patient) took responsibility for changing things. The specialist was matter-of-fact in tone and directed the discussion toward the issue the patient raised.

In the following example, a different technique is employed that deals with the same element of service—personal responsibility.

"Mrs. Prentice? I'm Miss Howard, with the Recreation Department. I just thought I'd stop by your room this afternoon and introduce myself. I'm usually in the lounge every evening, and I saw your name on the list of new residents last week, but you haven't been by, so I decided to come and see you."

"That's very nice of you. It is a little difficult for me to get around with my cane and all. I've been meeting a number of people since I arrived at the home. Miss Towsend, my social worker, has been here a few times, and took me around and introduced me to people. She hasn't been here in the evenings, so I guess that's why I haven't met you. Anyway, I usually go to bed after supper. I haven't been going out at night for a number of years."

"Oh, I'm sorry to hear that—we have a lot doing at Pine Manor in the evenings. There are concerts one night a week; a current events session (sometimes a visiting political candidate); two movies each week; some of the women make cookies and things; there is always a bridge game going; and one or the other of the club groups are meeting. Then there is the library, which is open until ten, and of course, the drama group practices, and then we have theater tours each month and the diners' club. Some people are working on a project concerning educational materials for retarded children. Oh, yes, there are many things to do in the evening."

"But I'm so old now. I used to do a lot of those things when I was younger. After my husband died, I sort of stopped doing a lot of things. My son and daughter-in-law took me out once in a while, but when they moved out of town, I had no one to take me any more. I decided with most of my friends dead too, or moved away, and the neighborhood changing so, there really was nothing much left for me. In fact, they are some of the reasons I decided to come to the Home. I might as well *give up* now as wait around a few more years!"

"Oh, I don't think you have to give up, and as for being younger, who do you think is doing all those things here at Pine Manor? How would it seem to you if I asked some of the other residents who have a special interest in certain activities to come and take you each evening to a different event; then after you have seen them all, and if nothing really interests you, I won't bother you again . . . but I'm sure you're going to find some things you'd like to do. This will only be for a week or so, and then it's up to you to decide what you want to do with your time."

In this second example, the specialist, although using a direct approach, offered support and encouragement. In addition, she presented a plan for continued support until Mrs. Prentice assumed responsibility for herself.

In the late 1950s, in the United States, a service was initiated in a large general hospital to help psychiatric patients assume personal responsibility for meeting their own need for recreation after discharge from the hospital. This service has become a model in many institutions.[1] Working as a team, the psychology department and the recreation department of the hospital joined forces with the municipal recreation department of the city in which the hospital was located. Prior to discharge, patients were counseled on an individual and group basis in the hospital regarding personal recreation responsibility, and then field trips were conducted by the municipal recreation staff to indicate adult recreation resources available in the community, and how these resources could be used.

In a recent study (1969) of recreation counseling practices, O'Morrow reported that over two-thirds of the 150 psychiatric institutions in the United States that offer recreation counseling service have as one of their objectives instruction of patients during the predischarge period—instruction calculated to teach them how to identify, locate, and use community recreation resources.[2] It is thought that this approach will assist the ex-patient, who has been dependent upon a "scheduled" recreation program within the institution over a period of time, to assume personal responsibility after discharge.

With regard to the second principal of *developing* a *personal philosophy of recreation appropriate to* one's *existential situation*, the therapeutic recreation specialist attempts to provide realistic information to the patient or client so that he may face reality. This is particularly important when he is faced with an altered life situation that dictates a change in leisure pattern.

> Miss Z., age 48, lives alone in a 4-room flat in a small building in a large city. Heart disease; essential hypertension (ordinary physical activity does not cause discomfort); retinopathy grade 2; bilateral myopic degeneration.
>
> Released from hospital to home care service. Visual acuity is poor and becoming progressively worse. Housekeeping service provided to clean, assist with shopping, prepare meals.

[1] W. E. Olsen and J. B. McCormack, "Recreation Counseling in the Psychiatric Service of A General Hospital," *Journal of Nervous and Mental Diseases*, CXXXV (April-June 1957), 237-39.

[2] G. S. O'Morrow, *A Study of Recreation Service to Psychiatric Patients in Relation to Pre-Discharge Planning and Aftercare* (New York: Teachers College, Columbia University, unpublished doctoral dissertation, 1969), p. 120.

Born in England, lived in the United States and Canada for 25 years. No relatives on this side of the Atlantic. Has made few friends or acquaintances over the years. Traveled extensively as a tutor in Germany, Italy, Switzerland, France, England. Always very active; played tennis, rode horseback, enjoyed swimming. A prolific reader, enjoyed theater and concerts.

Now spends most of time reminiscing, occasionally listens to radio, seldom attends church, a priest makes weekly visits to her home. She reports weakness, inability to see, only walks about three streets at a time when she goes out. Goes out some mornings for coffee in a nearby restaurant, enjoys talking with counterman and other customers. When weather permits, sits on bench near house in local park.

Asked if there is anything else she would like to do, she replied: "I'm content to sit in the sun. I'm really not interested in anything any more. After seven months of living like this, I feel there is not much more time left for me. It takes a long time to die though."

A series of interviews and weekly visits with the therapeutic recreation specialist was arranged for this patient when she attended the outpatient clinic. During the first session, she talked about things she used to enjoy, and felt that she would like to hear her favorite music more often. The specialist encouraged her in this, indicating that her disability did not preclude her owning a phonograph or tape recorder. In subsequent sessions this was discussed again, but this time the patient asked a number of practical questions regarding costs of equipment, the extent of her visual problem, and her limited ability with "gadgets and switches." The specialist answered her questions in a realistic manner, having precise information to give her. The patient asked the specialist to accompany her to purchase an inexpensive phonograph. They had talked about borrowing phonograph recordings from the public library, and the specialist introduced the patient to this procedure at another session.

After a few weeks, the patient was introduced to a local community recreation center close to her home where she could attend a public concert each month. At her second concert, she reported that she met some other ladies who were members of the center and who told her about a range of adult activities the center offered. The specialist encouraged the patient to join some of these activities, such as a great book discussion group, because the patient had had a lifelong interest in literature. She was introduced to the "talking book" concept, which allowed her to continue her interest in "reading" although her vision had prevented this.

Within a few more sessions, the patient reported that she had made some friends, and she was becoming involved in a number of activities. She said, "I thought I was too sick to do anything, and the end was near! I know I can't do most of what I used to do, but there are many things I can do, and I'm going to try to do them."

In this example, the specialist was rather successful, because it was obvious that there were many avenues open to the patient. Primarily the patient needed information and encouragement. The following example is in sharp contrast.

Mr. S., age 34, lives with wife in a 3-room street-level apartment in a public housing complex. Bilateral, above-the-knee amputee, confined to wheelchair; diabetes mellitus; diabetic angiopathy; arrested pulmonary tuberculosis. Mrs. S. is a registered nurse, attends out-patient clinic for follow-up of arrested tuberculosis. Both are unemployed. Possible Mr. S. has Buerger's disease, readmitted for work-up.

Mr. S. assists wife with housework, is able to go in and out without assistance. Helps some of the housing complex youngsters with their homework. Several afternoons, goes to the nearby park and "coaches" youngsters who play ball. Except for this activity and some shopping, Mr. and Mrs. S. seldom go out. At home, they watch TV, read, play cards and Scrabble.

In a preliminary interview with Mr. S. at the hospital, he reported that he would like to bowl, swim, do some woodwork, paint and "be social." He said he would like to take trips to public meetings, concerts, ball games, and would like to have a few days in the country each summer. He feels that he does not have access to adequate transportation and thus does not do these things. He cannot use public transportation, and cannot afford taxi service.

During a subsequent series of discussions with Mr. S., a number of factors were brough out in regard to his desires regarding recreation. It became explicit that because of his disability and his wife's situation, they could not possibly afford a recreation pattern such as he desired. He was using the lack of adequate transportation as a rationale, because even before his amputation he was not a very "social" person, did not go to concerts or public meetings, and the like. He was rather a lonely man, for whom youngsters took the place of adult friendship. He was encouraged to begin to do things with other adults at the hospital while he was there for the work-up. He met with the therapeutic recreation specialist a few more times; however, there seemed to be a regression to his previous pattern and little progress. At their last meeting, he said, "I've been thinking about calling the public recreation department and formally volunteering my services as a coach in the park. I can get there without any difficulty from our apartment, and the boys seem to like me, and they listen to what I say. Maybe when my wife and I get better, we can do some of the other things we have talked about."

It was unrealistic for Mr. S. to think of himself as a "volunteer" with the public recreation department—just as unrealistic as his notion that when his wife improved they would be able to engage in some of the recreation activities he talked about. It became apparent that Mr. S. had a number of emotional problems which prevented him from developing a personal philosophy of recreation that was realistic with regard to his situation, and before this could be done, he would need additional help. The specialist in this instance was not equipped to undertake this responsibility, and referred Mr. S. to the social work department of the hospital. Unlike the case of Miss Z., no amount of information and encouragement would alter Mr. S.'s perspective at this time.

Both of these principles—personal responsibility and an appropriate philosophy—are operant when a patient or client has reached a stage in life that might be described as a plateau. Generally, his mental health must be sound if he is to view the plateau with any degree of clarity. In the case of physical or intellectual impairment, he may or may not be aware of how this limits him. Part of the specialist's role is to help him understand this with respect to recreation participation—what types of activities and participations are within the realm of reality in spite of personal limitations, and what resources can be tapped for this purpose. Ultimately, the specialist is concerned with the patient's or client's ability to participate in recreative experience of his own choice, and to use recreation resources with a high degree of personal competence.

If the patient or client is still receiving active treatment, a variety of service elements can be introduced during this time which lead to education and information regarding personal responsibility and an appropriate philosophy.

Stimulation and Instruction

In addition to being aware of one's personal responsibility and holding an appropriate philosophy, a patient or client must perceive himself as a potentially active participant in the social and recreative life of his community, whether within the institution or outside it. To insure this type of perception, the therapeutic recreation specialist offers stimulation and instruction directed at three major concerns:

1. Improving general health and appearance.
2. Enhancing the self-image.
3. Minimizing atypical behavior.

The specialist will encourage patients or clients to be concerned with personal grooming, make suggestions about personal attributes which enhance their attractiveness, and indicate undesirable factors and behavior. He may schedule sessions in grooming for both men and women, keep a supply of sample items for resident use, enlist the aid of a volunteer for shopping excursions with regard to this element of service, or hold group and individual discussions with patients and clients regarding this issue. He may at times use a variety of resource personnel for this purpose, from his colleagues on an institutional staff to a range of personnel in the community. The following case material is illustrative of this element of service.

Progress note: Mr. T., Ward 6E

10/16 Patient came to lounge program. Tried to get other patients to interact with him. He was consistently rejected. He looked disheveled, pajamas and bathrobe dirty and creased, hair uncombed, perspiring profusely. He approached me, and body odor was oppressive. He left the lounge within a few minutes of his arrival.

10/17 Cleared with nursing staff re: Mr. T.'s personal appearance. Apparently no medical reason for this situation. Drug that he is taking may induce the perspiration. Stopped by his room and discussed this situation with him. Indicated that it would be preferable if he wore clean pajamas and bathed before he came to the lounge programs. Inquired if he had other pajamas and a comb. Promised to send him a sample deodorant.

10/20 Patient came to evening discussion group. He had on a new pair of pajamas, was clean, hair combed, and no evidence of body odor, although he still perspired. Observed that he used a handkerchief to absorb perspiration at this time. He participated in the discussion, and was not rejected by other patients. He stayed until the end of the session to ask about other programs.

The following is a short note from a community center report which deals with this element of service.

Worker report to supervisor, Young Adult Center, June 23.

Although it is obvious that little social dance skill has been taught to this group while they were at the State School, their cognitive condition does not preclude these learnings. They were quick to grasp a variety of dances, and the evening proved most successful. However, some problems do exist beyond their ability and capacity to dance. I had to spend some time with a few of the girls individually, discussing how they were dressed. A number of them wore too much make-up, which made them look grotesque. I would recommend that the Center sponsor a make-up and clothes workshop for these girls. Two or three sessions would be adequate. In addition, it appears that little attempt was made at the State School to indicate to the boys that a "girl is a gentle thing," since I found myself saying "take it easy" to a number of the boys after they learned the steps to a dance. Some of them are pretty rough. A third problem seems to be that JL is unaware of how seductive her behavior is. My co-worker and I agree that before the dance next Saturday night, one of us would talk with her about this. . . .

These two examples, in a general hospital and in a community center for mentally retarded adolescents, indicate the directness and appropriateness of this element of service. Judgments are based on a knowledge of behavioral norms operant in usual social situations of this type.

Manipulation of Resources

Although the manipulation of resources ultimately results in service to patients or clients, they are primarily indirect services. All therapeutic recreation specialists engage in this element of service to some degree; however, some specialists may find their major responsibility centered around one or two of the tasks that make up this element of service.

A. Community planning, development, and organization to enable persons with limitations to engage in recreative activity:

This task requires that a specialist working within a single institution or agency serve on an administrative committee within the setting—a committee concerned with the overall schedule, use of space and facilities, budget, and a host of other administrative factors. In some settings, responsibility may take the form of an interagency committee engaged in joint planning of the use of physical resources, transportation, or interpretation to public authorities or the public at large. This task may also take the form of a full-time position on the staff of a public or private agency (such as a municipal recreation department or a federation of health agencies) in which a specialist coordinates the use of numbers of public resources by individuals and groups who have limitations that affect their recreation participation. Usually, these resources are shared by persons who do not have such limitations.[3]

Generally, the tasks of persons who are concerned with community work fall into one of the following classifications:

1. Identifying, evaluating, defining needs of a community, or problems of a community;
2. Collecting appropriate factual data regarding community needs or problems;
3. Analyzing collected data, conducting secondary analysis of data from other sources, determining the implications of findings with regard to community needs or problems;
4. Determining appropriate and acceptable courses of action with respect to community needs and problems;
5. Activating and coordinating courses of action that the community deems necessary.

[3] See E. M. Avedon et al., *Activating Community Resources for Therapeutic Recreation Service* (New York: Comeback, Inc., 1966); W. W. Biddle, *Encouraging Community Development: Guide for Local Workers* (Toronto: Holt, Rinehart and Winston, Inc., 1968); W. W. Biddle, *The Community Development Process* (Toronto: Holt, Rinehart and Winston, Inc., 1965); R. Johns and D. F. DeMarche, *Community Organization and Agency Responsibility* (New York: Associaton Press, 1951); R. Robinson, *Serving the Small Community* (New York: Association Press, 1959); I. Sanders, *The Community: Introduction to a Social System* (New York, Ronald Press, 1966); V. M. Sieder, *The Rehabilitation Agency and Community Work* (Waltham, Mass.: Florence Heller Graduate School, 1966; R. L. Warren, *Studying Your Community* (New York: Russel Sage Foundation, 1955); and Youth and Recreation Branch, *Notes for Community Leaders* (Toronto: Ontario Department of Education, n.d.).

B. Administration and coordination of programs and services to enhance opportunities for recreative experiences for persons with limitations:

In a small institution, such as a nursing home, which houses approximately fifty persons, this task is a part of the specialist's total responsibility. In most instances however, administration and coordination of program services is usually a full-time responsibility in itself, whether it is in a specialized residential setting or a community-based agency program. Usually, a small agency cannot afford to maintain both administrative and leadership personnel for recreation service. However, the essential task of the administrator is the same whether he administers a program for 40 or 400 people. Difference is not in kind, but in degree. Some task variations exist with respect to the nature of the setting. As a consequence, some small agencies share personnel through the pooling of economic resources, and one administrator might administer a half-dozen small programs as a full-time position, while his counterpart in a large institution carries on the same tasks in a single setting.

A number of texts are available to personnel in the field of recreation regarding the process of administration, and thus little need be included here regarding this subject. However, it is important to indicate that in order to enhance opportunities for recreative experiences to persons with limitations, considerable attention must be paid by the administrator to agency policy.

Although the *philosophy* of a setting concerns its orientation, its values, and its goals, the *policy* is the broad general guide to action that is established to achieve these values and goals. *Procedures* are the specific measures used to carry out policy.

Policy is a settled or determined course of action adapted by a governing body or an individual, but it should not be an immutable law or rigid set of rules. Policy indicates a settled course of action—a course that can be changed with the times. When decisions made are contrary to policy, this may mean a need for a policy change. Deviations are a turning away from the old way of doing things and should not be considered just momentary exceptions to the general rule. Deviations from policy should be made only with a full determination that a new way is distinctly better than an older way. Policy enables staff to maintain a sense of direction.

Thus a new administrator of a therapeutic recreation program would be interested in understanding how policies are made in his setting, who makes them, and the circumstances under which they can be changed. He must also determine how policy change will affect service to patients and clients, to others in the setting, and to the community at large. Usually, policy in therapeutic recreation service is part of a mosaic of broad institutional policies, and alterations in one aspect of the mosaic affects the total mosaic.

Another difficult aspect of administration in therapeutic recreation service in a setting concerned with a primary mission other than recreation is the matter of expenditure. The nature of a recreation program budget eludes most fiscal control officers in these settings. When they examine sample budgets from texts concerned with the administration of recreation service, they find that these are exemplary of large municipal agencies and include many items not normally found in a therapeutic recreation program budget. Also, they find that many items that are included cannot be found in sample operating budgets. To alleviate this situation, the following accounting scheme for a therapeutic recreation department in a multiservice setting is offered. This scheme includes accounting codes, examples of typical expenditure types, and explanations as required; it must be translated into accounting units by the administrator, based upon frequency of service, size of staff, and number of program participants.

ACCOUNTING SCHEME FOR CLASSIFICATION OF EXPENDITURES INCURRED IN A PROGRAM OF RECREATION SERVICE WITHIN A MULTISERVICE SETTING

The following suggested scheme is exemplary, and is intended to serve as a model. It is by no means exhaustive, and the user is encouraged to adapt or modify it to suit his particular needs. It is assumed that the sponsoring agency maintains a much more comprehensive account procedure relative to the multiplicity of services offered. This suggested scheme concerns only those expenditures incurred through the provision of a program of recreation service.

ACCOUNT	EXPENDITURE	EXPLANATION
1000	Personnel expenditure and related expense	
1100	regular full-time employees	salaries
1200	regular part-time employees	salaries
1300	regular full-time employees	wages
1400	temporary employees	wages
1500	entertainers	fees
1600	consultants	fees
1700	personnel benefits	insurance
1800	education benefits	tuition
1900	other compensations	
2000	Purchase of service	(contract or fee)
2100	Communication	
2110	telephone and telegraph	
2120	postage	
2130	messenger service	
2200	Transportation	
2210	hired drivers	owned car

Elements of Service: Part I

ACCOUNT	EXPENDITURE	EXPLANATION
2220	hired vehicles	
2230	transport service	
2240	local public transport	
2250	railroad & bus	staff meet
2260	airline & transfers	staff meet
2270	storage & parking	owned car
2280	mileage & tolls	
2300	Subsistence	(lodging, meals)
2310	staff conference per diem	
2320	subsistence of other than staff	
2330	care of pets	
2400	Repairs	
2410	television sets	agency-owned
2420	motion-picture equipment	
2430	audio equipment	phonograph, etc.
2440	power tools, etc.	garden, craft
2450	owned vehicles	
2460	other equipment	
2470	musical instruments	
2500	Utilities	
2600	Janitorial	(special charges)
2700	Processing services	
2710	printing and binding	
2720	duplicating	(e.g., Xerox)
2730	photographic services	
2740	advertising and publication	
2750	data processing	
2800	Rental of motion pictures	
2900	Piano tuning	
3000	Commodities	
3100	Supplies—	items consumed or used up
3110	stationery & related consumable supplies	
3120	duplication & mimeographing	
3130	food products	
3140	gasoline and oil, etc.	
3150	party decorations	
3160	recording supplies—tapes, records	
3170	books, magazines, newspapers, etc.	
3180	games, cards, music, related supplies	
3190	prizes, gifts, etc.	

ACCOUNT	EXPENDITURE	EXPLANATION
3200	Materials—	items converted to other uses
3210	wood and related products	
3220	clay and related products	
3230	metal and metal products	
3240	paints and related products	
3250	fibers, wools, woven goods, etc.	
3260	hides, pelts, leather, etc.	
3270	glass, plastic, etc.	
3280	other materials	
4000	Properties	(owned by the agency)
4100	Equipment	
4110	furniture, carts, etc.	
4120	hand tools (craft and garden)	
4130	power tools and accessories	
4140	musical instruments	
4150	television equipment	
4160	audio equipment	
4170	office equipment	
4180	library equipment	
4190	other equipment	
4200	Facilities	(other than general agency)
4210	trees, plants, etc.	
4220	improvements	(e.g., stage lighting)
5000	Charges	
5100	Equipment rental	
5110	audiovisual	
5120	tools and related	
5130	office machinery	
5200	Facility rental	
5210	swimming pool	
5220	bowling alley	
5230	campsite	
5240	other	
5300	Admissions	(theater, sporting events, etc.)
5400	Insurance	
5500	Registrations	
5600	Subscriptions and publications	

(C) Consultation to other professional persons to promote and expand recreative opportunities for persons with limitations:

Elements of Service: Part I

This task may take two major forms. A staff member whose primary role might be administrative or leadership may be asked to offer consultation to another staff member regarding service to a patient or client. Consultation is the process by which a professional person interacts with another professional person in order to enable the latter to enhance his functioning to his service recipients. Thus, a nurse, physician, teacher, or social worker might seek consultation with a therapeutic recreation specialist regarding service to a specific patient or client. The second form of consultation is a full-time responsibility. In this form, a therapeutic recreation specialist functions as a consultant focusing upon program development, staff education, and administrative interpretation. Some of these personnel are employed by regional agencies such as a state, provincial, or county health department; a recreation department; or in larger municipalities by coordinating agencies of nonprofit or church auspices.

DEFINING CONSULTATION

Consultation is an interactive process that takes place between two professional persons—the consultant and the consultee. In the interaction, the consultant *attempts* to help the consultee solve a problem, clarify an issue concerning the setting in which the consultee practices, helps introduce a new service or modify an old service, or engages in special tasks such as in-service education or research. While the consultant is helping the consultee in dealing with the presenting situation, he is also educating him to be able to function in future situations without assistance.

Consultation is an indirect rather than a direct service to a patient or client, and is generally offered to professional personnel in key administrative and supervisory positions first in order to maximize the effect. Meetings are usually held at the consultee's place of work rather than at the consultant's office. The consultation relationship is usually fully confidential to insure trust of the consultee and to prevent disruption of agency-community relationships. Consultants do not generally see a client or a patient except in the company of the consultee in order to demonstrate a principle or enhance the consultation relationship.

The process of consultation is sometimes confused with other roles operant in work with patients and clients; namely psychotherapy, supervision, administration, and collaboration. The following presents some similarities and differences:

> PSYCHOTHERAPY—an explicit contract between therapist and patient in which therapist takes responsibility for attempting to help patient solve *personal* problems, working with whatever feelings or experiences are of concern to patient; CONSULTATION—a contract between consultant and consultee to provide assistance with a *work* problem that agency presents to consultee; consultant does *not* attempt to resolve intrapsychic problems.

SUPERVISION—supervisor prepared in same field as supervisee, has responsibility to oversee work of supervisee, is responsible for supervisee's performance, deals directly when it does not meet certain expectations, rates performance, recommends promotion, increments, and discharge; CONSULTATION—not vested with or assuming such responsibility; in some situations does not know consultee's field of competence, consultee free to accept or reject consultant's suggestions, consultant not responsible for the consultee's effectiveness.

ADMINISTRATION—concerned with efficient execution of agency policy, budgetary and personnel considerations basic to program implementation; CONSULTATION—not responsible for program effectiveness or agency policy, although may contribute toward change or strengthening of policy and program.

COLLABORATION—interaction between two or more professional persons of similar or different preparation who contribute (from the framework of their professional competence) information and experience that helps to solve a *common* professional problem—they may follow through on a joint activity; CONSULTATION—consultee asks consultant to help, consultant not expected to implement or act in behalf of consultee.

FRAME OF REFERENCE

Certain theoretical principles are adhered to by many consultants. Some of these principles are as follows:

—General questions put to the consultant are converted into appropriate specific situations for most effective use of the consultant's time;
—Whenever possible, the consultant permits the consultee to solve his own problems, and supports or reinforces his judgment, if thought sound;
—Although the process affords the opportunity for change, the decision for change always rests with the consultee;
—The consultant avoids contributing to the diffusion of the professional role of the consultee;
—The consultant is not responsible for the professional adequacy of the consultee.

Although some operating agencies employ a person whom they call a consultant, they expect him to play a nonconsultation role. In effect, what they seek is a "facilitator," "monitor," "mediator," or perhaps "investigator."

Generally consultants play the same role, regardless of the presenting situation, or whether the task is in the area of planning, policy, recruitment, in-service education, operating efficiency, personnel use, problem-solving, program evaluation, community resource use, or others. From a sociological perspective, all consultants are interested in a setting as a "formal organization," because concern is with the ecological, structural, and procedural aspects of the agency or institution. From an ecological point of view, a consultant wants to

Elements of Service: Part I

know how the agency or institution relates to society. From a structural point of view, he wants to know what are the agency's stated purposes, explicit rules, defined roles, norms, and goals of its system, informal deviations in the system, status of functionaries, and the like. From a procedural frame of reference, he looks for the factors of change and decision-making, who are the influentials in the setting, how they relate to the power groups, and what are the reference groups for the setting. In examining the setting, the consultant is concerned with whether the service recipients use the setting because they have a like set of values or because they are a "physical locality grouping." The consultant is also interested in the life style of the consultee group and whether this group is a subcultural group which has no new "inputs" to speak of. A consultant tries to determine who really has the power to act when there is a problem.

Consultants are aware that their value systems and that of consultees differ. Each has his own set of "macro inputs"—such as professional identity, political party, and the like. However, the consultee also has "micro inputs"—such as staff and local reference groups, factors of promotion, status, and the like. When consultants direct efforts at innovations in a part of a social system, this will affect the entire system and consequently the "micro inputs" of the consultee.

Consultants are primarily change agents who focus upon goals, convictions, beliefs, attitudes, insights, behavior, methods, techniques, program content, and so forth. Change in these factors can occur when the consultant has been able to establish a good relationship with the consultee, when the consultee does not support or reinforce the present situation, and when the consultant offers an alternative course of action. As a consequence, the result may be change, change and regression, or no change.

From a psychological perspective, it is apparent that the consultant is an "outsider" stepping into a "closed system." As a result, he faces a number of problems until he can overcome this situation. Consultees often consider the consultant to be an expert in his field. The consultant may or may not be. Often the consultant is more experienced than the consultee, and perhaps because he does not have a vested interest in the situation he can listen more carefully and weigh the facts more accurately. Because of this "outsider-expert" image, some consultees fear a consultant, others become impotent, and still others use their energies to prove their adequacy. Once the consultant can do away with this image, he can enable the consultee to redirect his energy to the situation at hand. In reality, most solutions to presenting situations are in the settings themselves. The function of the consultant may be only to reinforce solutions already proposed, introduce new information regarding solutions, or raise issues that have not been made explicit in the setting.

SOME CONSULTATION ERRORS

The following are examples of errors in technique that foster relationship problems between the consultant and the consultee. These problems often end in termination of the consultation relationship.[4]

—Offering advice or solutions too readily or quickly without giving the consultee a chance to use his own skills; or remaining verbally inactive over a sequence of sessions, offering the consultee no opportunity to benefit from the sessions.
—Commenting on too many areas of interaction in a given session in such a way as to either burden the consultee or compound his insecurity; or permitting the consultation to go everywhere and encompass everything, or overdirecting the process, or keeping it so narrow that it becomes nonproductive.
—Not listening for the central issue, so that the content can be fairly specific; or becoming a protagonist for one's own point of view, or introducing one's own biases inappropriately.
—Conveying the notion or assuming the position of expert in an area of the consultee's professional competence when it is different from one's own area of competence; lacking awareness of one's own limitations, and promoting the illusion of omnipotence.
—Assuming there is need to help the consultee with "everything" he brings to the consultation session; or when resolution of conflict (either explicitly or implicity) diffuses the consultee's professional role.

SOME GENERAL ACTIVITIES OF CONSULTANTS

I. Developing a plan for consultation
   A. Elicit preliminary information concerning the purpose of the consultation from the consultee;
   B. Interpret the consultant's role in relation to the purpose of the consultation to the consultee;
   C. Arrange time and meeting place at the convenience of the consultee;
   D. Present a preliminary plan related to the needs of the consultee and the time that is available;
   E. State fees and charges when indicated.
II. Preparing for the consultation
   A. Gather information from available resources that bears upon the consultation;
   B. Elicit specific information from the consultee in relation to the situation;
   C. Evaluate the information.
III. Establishing a relationship with the consultee
   A. Encourage free expression of ideas and feelings;
   B. Create a permissive atmosphere for discussion;
   C. Interact in a realistic manner;
   D. Listen to the consultee.

[4] V. Kazanjian, S. Stein, and W. L. Weinberg, *Introduction to Mental Health Consultation*, U.S. Public Health Service Publication No. 922, 1962, p. 9.

Elements of Service: Part I

IV. Clarifying goals and defining issues
   A. Encourage objective and realistic discussion of the situation;
   B. Summarize and pinpoint significant factors;
   C. Analyze aspects of the situation.
V. Giving pertinent information and ideas
   A. Make available knowledge and skills of experts;
   B. Discuss adaptations and resources as indicated;
   C. Demonstrate appropriate methods and skills.
VI. Focusing the consultation
   A. Use periodic summaries (written or oral) as a directing force;
   B. Clarify important aspects of the situation.
VII. Formulating courses of action
   A. Discuss potentialities and limitations of the situation;
   B. Identify realistic alternatives or new directions;
   C. Evaluate course of action.
VIII. Selecting a course of action
   A. Assist the consultee to select action directed toward the achievement of desired goals;
   B. Indicate that the selection of a course of action must be the decision of the consultee if it is to be effectively implemented;
   C. Help the consultee to arrive at a decision that is a genuine expression of will.
IX. Promoting self-direction in implementation of action
   A. Instill confidence in the consultee's own ability;
   B. Promote psychological readiness in the consultee to assume responsibility.
X. Planning further consultation if indicated
   A. Assure the consultee of continued interest;
   B. Suggest other resources for consultation.
XI. Preparing a report of the consultation
   A. Describe and interpret the content of the consultation;
   B. Evaluate the effectiveness of the consultation.
XII. Terminating the consultation relationship
   A. Furnish reports, documents, and final correspondences as indicated;
   B. Render a bill for services, if indicated.

D. Survey and elimination of social barriers preventing persons with limitations from engaging in recreative experience:

This task may be performed by a therapeutic recreation specialist who is part of a professional organization that has taken this task on as an organizational responsibility, or it may be engaged in by a specialist as a regular function with regard to the setting in which he is employed. Employment, for example, may be in a nonprofit health agency that serves children with neurological limitations. The task of the specialist may be to determine which local recreation resources can be used by children served by the agency. The specialist may find in his survey that many resources could be used if there were some modifications in the attitude of the administrative authority controlling a given resource, or if there were some architectural modifications to the resources.

Potential recreation participants who have limited physical ability have some of the following problems:

LIMITATION IN WALKING

—Difficulty in walking distances because of muscle weakness caused by disease or age;
—Difficulty in walking on nonlevel and nonsmooth surfaces because of (1) reliance upon braces, crutches, prosthesis; (2) cardiac, pulmonary, or neurological problems that affect strength, flexibility, and coordination; (3) sensory impairment affecting balance; or (4) impairment of joints;
—Inability to walk but can propel themselves in a wheelchair on level and certain graded surfaces;
—Inability to propel a wheelchair because of extensive impairment and must be accompanied by an attendant.

LIMITATIONS IN SEEING AND/OR HEARING

—Difficulty in seeing and/or hearing warnings and safety hazards because of limited vision or audition due to impairment or age;
—Inability to see and/or hear warnings and safety hazards because of extensive impairment.

LIMITATION IN USE OF HANDS AND ARMS

—Difficulty in opening gates or doors, manipulating equipment, etc., because of muscle or joint weakness or because of the necessity of manipulating crutches, a cane, or a wheelchair;
—Inability to open gates or doors, etc., because of extensive impairment in the muscles and joints of the hands and arms.

LIMITATION IN UNDERSTANDING INFORMATION

—Difficulty in reading printed signs indicating directions, warnings, etc., because of partial sight or moderate intellectual limitations;
—Inability to read printed signs because of blindness or severe intellectual limitations.

As a consequence, a number of resources are now available to assist the specialist in adapting recreation resources to meet the needs of persons who have special needs.[5] The resource in question may be a neighborhood playground,

---

[5] See Architectural Barriers Commission Publications, Rehabilitation Services Administration, U.S. Department of Health, Education and Welfare, Washington, D.C.; also, American Standards Association, *Specifications for Making Buildings and Facilities Accessible to and Usable by the Physically Handicapped* (New York: The Association, 1961); S. Goldsmith, *Designing for the Disabled: A Manual of Technical Information*

and the playground supervisor feels that children with coordination problems are a hazard on the playground. The specialist would then embark upon the task of educating this supervisor to allay his fears, and indicate how these children might benefit from this experience and not cause a hazardous situation. In addition, this same playground may have a toilet which, because of the way it has been built, becomes unusable by a child with a coordination problem. The specialist would indicate this problem, and point out how a slight modification, such as a grab-bar, would eliminate this barrier. Perhaps the situation is further complicated by parents of nondisabled children who object to their children playing with a disabled child. The specialist in this instance may meet with these parents and discuss the situation, helping them to alter their objections.

E. Modification and adaptation of facilities, equipment, transportation, and other resources that have potential recreative value to persons who have limitations:

This task is usually performed by specialists having direct leadership responsibility with patients and clients; however, there are some people who engage in this task exclusively on a full-time basis. In this latter instance, they are concerned with not only potential recreative resources, but all resources involved in daily living. Often these modifications may be rather simple but ingenious, such as using an old-fashioned scrubbing brush as a card holder for someone who can't use both hands but would like to continue to play bridge; or substituting spring-clip clothespins for checkers and modifying the board with pegs instead of a flat playing surface so someone who has a problem grasping and releasing the flat checkers can still play this game. Other modifications may be more elaborate, such as some of the sports adapted for wheelchair players, or devices that allow persons with manual limitations to continue to be creative in an art activity, or the large-print materials and compensating devices for older persons with visual limitations. The most comprehensive catalog of modified recreation equipment is found in E. Lowman and J. L. Klinger's *Aids to Independent Living* (New York: McGraw-Hill, 1969), pp. 566-646. This volume includes a range of materials from table games to gardening and sport supplies, as well as information concerning transportation, dress, and the like.

In a number of nations today special centers have been developed for this purpose. In England, The Disabled Living Foundation offers special materials on a variety of recreation related subjects. In Sweden, Denmark, and The

(London: Royal Institute of British Architects Technical Information Service, 1963); *National Building Code, Building Standards for the Handicapped* (Ottawa, Canada: National Research Council, 1965); H. Rusalem et al., "Architectural Barriers to the Participation of Disabled Persons in Community Recreation Activities," *Journal of Chronic Disease* Vol XVIII (1965), 161-66.

Netherlands special centers not only furnish materials but display modified equipment, demonstrate its use, and conduct research into needs for new adaptations. With the advent of transistors and printed circuts have come a host of ingenious equipment modifications. For example, an agency for the blind in Yugoslavia has introduced a chess set which audibly announces the name of the piece you have touched, and the space it is on, then the space that it is moved to. The set can be altered to respond in German, French, English, or Serbo-Croatian at this time!

F. Research and development of new methods for delivering service to persons who are limited:

As in the case of many other tasks, this element of service may be part of the total responsibility of a therapeutic recreation specialist in a direct service setting, or it may occupy the specialist full-time. This task may assume simple proportions, such as recording responses to a given activity over a period of time in a long-term care setting as a basis for program improvement, or it may become an elaborate project involving a sophisticated research design which includes staff observers, TV monitors, and advanced statistical analysis of data. Some research is quite pragmatic and of an action nature, such as the development of methods for strengthening independent participation of blind persons in community recreation programs. In contrast, and more esoteric, is research concerned with such factors as the relationship between bleeding episodes in hemophilia and emotional factors generated in competitive games. Some research may be of an administrative nature, such as determining effective staffing and organizational patterns in various settings, or an assessment of the economic benefits of offering specific services in a given setting. Other research may be of a clinical nature and involve participation in a project designed to develop methods for incorporating recreative techniques into a care program that is determining ways to retard progressive neurological deterioration. Still other types of research may be conducted away from clinical practice and involve such techniques as secondary analysis of comparative data, logical inference methods, and historical and documentary analysis.[6]

G. Education of persons to provide therapeutic recreation service:

In every profession, not only do college and university personnel engage in this task on a full-time basis but all practitioners have a responsibility to carry on and assist in the education of personnel. Thus, administrative and supervisory

---

[6] See E. M. Avedon, "The Role of Research In Health-Oriented Recreation Service," *Recreation Research: Collected Papers* (Washington, D.C.: National Education Association, 1966), pp. 18-24; and E. M. Avedon, "Some Thoughts On Research and Therapeutic Recreation Service," *Recreation in Treatment Centers* (Washington, D.C.: National Recreation and Park Association, 1967), Vol. VI.

Elements of Service: Part I 75

personnel conduct in-service education programs with their own staff, and often offer practical experiences to students in pre-service education programs. Consultants and others permit pre-service personnel to engage in observation and lecture as clinical affiliates in pre-service classes. In addition to involvement in professional education within their own profession, therapeutic recreation specialists engage in training courses for sub-professional personnel and volunteers, as well as student nurses, interns, administrators, and others.

Another aspect of this element of service is the sharing of information, theories, concepts, research findings, and reports with one's colleagues and co-workers. This is usually done through the publication of articles, monographs, and books. Retrieval of published information in therapeutic recreation service has not been an easy task. Dr. F. W. Martin, who established TRIC (Therapeutic Recreation Information Center), a computerized information retrieval process, explains why this is so and what is needed to remedy this situation.

Information Sources F.W. Martin*

The ideal point in time to begin the development of an information system would be that moment when the first traces of information related to a field or discipline began to enter the mainstream of knowledge. Every increment of time thereafter represents an increase in the cost factor for retrieval of information already produced and a percentage loss of information that will probably never be retrieved.

Unless the origins of a field or discipline have some dramatic or historically significant beginning, they will usually be cloaked with vagueness or entwined in conflicting ex post facto interpretations. Therapeutic recreation service cannot claim any special historic beginnings, therefore, along with many others, it must endure the alternative. Consequently, information system development for the field of therapeutic recreation service follows a period of historical activity which can be expected to exert a variety of influences on the document production of this service area.

The *practice* of therapeutic recreation service has been traced to periods as early as the fourth century *B.C.* Many persons in the field locate the organization of *professional* recreation service for ill and disabled persons during World War II. Within the United States, The American Recreation Society formally recognized the concept of *hospital recreation* by establishing a special section within this organization to represent concerned personnel as early as 1949. The American Association for Health, Physical Education, and Recreation supported a concept of *recreation therapy* by using this label for special sectional meetings in the early 1950s. The merging and expansion of these concepts to include all areas of disability resulted in the introduction of the concept of

---

* Reprinted by permission of the author.

therapeutic recreation in the late 1950s. Primarily as a result of the activity of concerned organizations such as Comeback, Inc., the concept of therapeutic recreation received sufficient support so that with the merger of several professional organizations into the National Recreation and Park Association in 1966, the professional sub-section of the NRPA designated to represent professionals engaged in the delivery of service to ill and disabled persons was called the National Therapeutic Recreation Society.

The journal of the National Association of Recreation Therapists (another organization which merged into the NRPA) was called *Recreation for the Ill and Handicapped.* This journal was soon retitled *Therapeutic Recreation Journal.* In 1970, the annual published by the National Therapeutic Recreation Society (NTRS) *Recreation in Treatment Centers* was similarly retitled *Therapeutic Recreation Annual.* This act almost completed the process of identification by persons in recreation service to the ill and disabled with the concept of Therapeutic Recreation Service as a generic reference to a number of specialized recreation activities within the framework of the disabled and the disadvantaged. Some institutions remain attached to earlier concepts and continue to refer to their programs in this area as hospital or institutional recreation. In some places the adjective "medical" is used, ignoring the scope of practice.

During the historical development of therapeutic recreation service, the general field of recreation also experienced developmental changes. From a primary concern focusing on play behavior and facilities for children and youth, the recreation field expanded its concerns to include service to all age groups in a variety of settings. It is currently experiencing an intensive concern with regard to the concept of *leisure* and its relevance to the general human conditon. The titling of the NRPA Journal *The Journal of Leisure Research,* and a variety of other publications since 1971, reflect this intensified focus. Insofar as the field of therapeutic recreation service is a subsection of the general field, its literature can be expected to react to such influences.

Diversity of Information Sources

The historical developments of the field of therapeutic recreation service have contributed to a literature related to the delivery of service to the ill and disabled that is scattered throughout a diverse collection of document sources. Because the *practice* of recreation service for ill and disabled persons considerably preceded the development of an organized *professional* service, other outlets for reporting this activity were needed. Medicine, Nursing, Rehabilitation, Education, Religion, Social Work, Corrections, and others have been concerned with and, at one time or another, have influenced the development of recreation service in this area of practice. In the process they have contributed to its literature, both in the publications identified with those service areas and in the publications that subsequently emerged from the professionalization of this service.

The diffusion of the literature of therapeutic recreation service explains in part the high frequency of documents concerning therapeutic recreation in non-recreation source periodicals. In addition to the large input of documents from recreation publications, *Mental Retardation Abstracts, Rehabilitation Literature,* and *Psychological Abstracts* contribute a significantly large portion of meaningful, related content to the literature.

Medlars, a computerized information retrieval system in the field of health-related services, is the largest single secondary source of documents concerning therapeutic recreation service.

The following primary and secondary U.S. sources have revealed the highest frequency of source potential for documents revelant to therapeutic recreation service:

Primary Recreation Sources

Therapeutic Recreation Journal
Parks and Recreation
ICRH Newsletter
Therapeutic Recreation Annual
Journal of Health, Physical Education, and Recreation

Other Primary Sources

Nursing Times
Nursing Mirror
Journal of Rehabilitation
Hospital and Community Psychiatry
American Journal of Nursing
Journal of the American Geriatric Society

Secondary Sources

Medlars
Mental Retardation Abstracts
Rehabilitation Literature
Psychological Abstracts

Systematic searching of the primary and secondary sources indicated above should result in high retrieval efficiency in relation to searching time and cost factors for information relevant to the delivery of therapeutic recreation service. It cannot be assumed that other information sources, both primary and secondary, will not yield high frequencies of document references relevant to therapeutic recreation service. Changes in indexing strategies, journals covered in search strategies, and other factors can easily be varied to have a greater sensitivity for the documents of the therapeutic recreation service area. Continual examination of potential information sources in spite of low yield expectations should be a function of an ongoing system in order to be in a position to react to such changes.

The following illustrate some of the problems inherent in utilization of titles alone in information retrieval.

Toby Levinson and G. Sereny, (Toronto, Ontario: Donwood Foundation), "An Experimental Evaluation of Insight Therapy for the Chronic Alcoholic," *Canadian Psychiatric Association Journal,* 14 (2) (1969), 143-146. Sixty alcoholics beyond the acute withdrawal phase spent six weeks in a continuing care unit where they participated in one of two programs. Program A consisted of regular psychiatrically oriented treatment with a well-balanced, well-structured program including didactic lectures, films, community meetings, occupational therapy, group psychotherapy, and *recreational* activity. Program B discontinued formal aspects, and subjects were encouraged to use occupational and recreational facilities, with the responsibility for seeking help placed on the subject. Results showed 28 percent of the psychological treatment group improved, and 31 percent of the recreational group improved. It is concluded that in dealing with this particular patient, a treatment program emphasizing *recreation* is at least as effective and in fact may be even more effective than a program geared toward establishing psychological insights.

Bernard A. Stotsky and Joan R. Dominick, (Northeaster University, College of Educaton) "Mental Patients in Nursing Homes: 1. Social Deprivation and Regression," *Journal of the American Geriatrics Society,* 17 (1) (1969), 33-34. Made a one-year controlled study of sixteen nursing homes containing 1400 patients to determine the effects of therapeutic activities in these settings. Deprivation in nursing homes was found to be related to lack of *recreation* and occupational therapy, space for group socialization and activities, and a common dining room. Also related were the absence of volunteer workers, separation of subjects on different floors, and minimal socialization between male and female patients. Case reports are presented. Proposed programs for overcoming these problems are discussed.

Neither of the citations in the two document references above (from *Psychological Abstracts*) specifically mention therapeutic recreation in any way. However, an examination of the abstracts (emphasis added) clearly reveals that some form of recreation service is a variable in both instances.

Terminology

The diffusion of relevant document sources, competing threads of historical development, and the relative youthfulness of this service profession have served to generate almost as much confusion as order regarding its terminology.

From the name of the field itself, which competing factions would prefer to see labeled differently, to specific service areas served by the field, such as mental retardation, brain-injured, aging, and the like, terminology is applied in what appears to be an almost random fashion to concepts, in spite of other terms already assigned to the same concept. Reacting in what appears to be a kind of frustration related to some of the terminology confusion of the field, the United States Veteran's Administration has labeled its recreation personnel *Therapeutic Recreation Therapists.*

Controversies have also appeared in the literature of therapeutic recreation service in relation to the interaction between label and concept. One of these has been the issue proposed by interchangeable use of the words "disabled" and "handicapped." In spite of some cogent arguments expressed regarding semantic differences between the two, the word "handicapped" is seemingly so entrenched in popular usage and even within professional circles that the use of the two labels applied to the same concept will probably continue.

Competing classification systems in fields served by therapeutic recreation specialists have produced some interesting terminological problems. It has been reported that eleven different classification systems have been utilized at some time or other, and several simultaneously, to describe intellectually impaired persons. These include such words as "educable," "trainable," "custodial," along with "borderline," "mild," "moderate," "severe," and "profound" as examples. Thus, until some consistency in the use of terminology develops and there is relative agreement regarding classifications and labels in the field of therapeutic recreation service, the retrieval of information will remain a complex problem for the average practitioner as well as for the specialist.

7
Elements of Service
Part II

Activity Programming

There are five major elements of service concerned with the conduct of activity. Uninformed persons, on viewing recreaton personnel conducting activity programs for persons who may be ill, disabled, or institutionalized, tend to think of these programs only as a source of fun for participants, and often question their inclusion in a treatment milieu. They do not consider this aspect of service as a part of a care plan or goal orientation of the setting, but tend to view it as a humanitarian effort, or what is worse, as a luxurious anachronism.

On the contrary, when a therapeutic recreation specialist involves a patient or client in an activity, it is related to the reason for which the person is present in the setting. Which aspect of activity programming is employed in each participant's situation depends upon the knowledge and skill of the specialist, the type of setting, the nature of the treatment or care plan, and the established activity program within the setting. Involving a patient or client in an activity program is not based on the notion that "everyone needs recreation." Although this may be true, everyone does not need an *organized* recreation program. Nor is involvement based on the notion of "as long as you've nothing better to do...". At times "nothing" may be better than "something," and "nothing" may be the treatment of choice.

Activity involvement is usually encouraged in relation to one of the following five objectives:

    1. Diagnosis and Evaluation

Elements of Service: Part II

2. Treatment and Care Plans
3. Altered Life Situation
4. Predischarge Counseling
5. Sheltered Experience

Programming for Diagnostic and Evaluation Purposes

There is nothing mystical or magical about the process of diagnosis or evaluaton—however, it must be accurate because treatment and care plans are based upon the results of the diagnostic or evaluation process. Generally, in a medical setting, a physician is responsible for coordinating the diagnostic process, utilizing the process to arrive at a diagnosis, and ultimately to establish a treatment plan. Information required by a physician is of various kinds; for example, laboratory reports, test reports, clinical reports, medical history, and others. In a nursing home or other long-term care setting, nursing personnel may have similar responsibility with regard to a care plan, while in a social agency, social diagnosis is the responsibility of a social worker. In a school for the mentally retarded, an educator often has this responsibility, and in a correctional institution, a correctional specialist or criminologist engages in evaluation to develop a rehabilitation plan. In a vocational rehabilitation setting, evaluation is conducted by a vocational counselor. In all of these settings and others, recreation personnel can assist in providing data that will complement and supplement the work of other professional persons contributing to a diagnostic or evaluation process.

Recreation personnel bring a special perspective to each setting because their focus is upon expected social behavior in social situations. Educational and experiential preparation sensitizes them to individual differences within a range of expected social behaviors. In addition, they are cognizant of a variety of usual behavioral responses to popular recreation activities. This awareness allows them to recognize unusual reactions or disequilibrium.

Although most personnel in special settings are often pathologically oriented, recreation personnel tend to focus on healthy aspects of personality. This focus usually concerns the individual in group social situations of an informal nature rather than a structured one-to-one relationship in a formal atmosphere. It should also be recognized that the contribution of a recreation specialist to the diagnostic and evaluaton process may be a subtle one, and may be quite minimal, depending upon the situation, the setting, and the person concerned. For example, on a playground, if a child begins to break out in spots or starts to cough or sneeze continually, the only contribution to the diagnostic process a recreation specialist might make is to state that he had not observed this phenomena earlier in the activity period. If the child was a frequent participant, the specialist might add that this phenomena was not observed previously.

A general contribution that a therapeutic recreation specialist can make to the diagnostic or evaluation process is visual observation of physical changes during activity participation. Each set of changes has meaning for the person coordinating the diagnostic or evaluation process. The recreation specialist should be aware that a particular set of behavior signs may reveal a specific disorder, and should be reported. For example, while conducting a game night in a senior center, a specialist reported the following:

> Mr. S. was playing poker, and was holding three queens. As one of the other players exposed his hand at the end of the game and revealed three kings, Mr. S. began to exhibit shortness of breath, his complexion began taking on a bluish tinge, and then he fainted.

In a school for the deaf, a recreation specialist reported

> John R. consistently attends my morning craft class. His face always seems to be "puffy" and his eyelids appear swollen. When he comes to my evening hobby group, his face isn't puffy. Curiously enough, he complains that he has difficulty standing in the evenings at the lathe for long periods of time, indicating that his ankles and feet swell up.

When a participant attends an activity session consistently, the recreation specialist forms a mental set regarding the participant's usual appearance and behavior. If he notes some change, this may have significance and should be reported.

It is expected that all members of an institutional staff would report information of a physical nature such as the following:

1. Reported visual or auditory disturbances;
2. Indications that the participant is in pain—constant, intermittent, dull, etc.;
3. An unusual lack of energy;
4. Relatively severe itching, tenderness, swelling;
5. Apparent change in skin color and tone—bluish, reddish, whitish, wetness, dryness, clamminess;
6. Severe change in respiration, causing discomfort;
7. Unusually uncoordinated and clumsy behavior;
8. Complaints of weakness and numbness;
9. Rapid mood changes;
10. An abrupt change in participant behavior that is inconsistent with previous behavior.

However, general physical changes or information about them is not the major contribution of personnel in therapeutic recreation to the diagnostic or evaluation process, but rather behavioral information of a social nature gathered during an interview or activity.

Generally, the information the therapeutic recreation specialist contributes to the diagnostic and evaluation process is quite specific, and includes the following:

1. INTERVIEW[1]

It is preferable to interview a patient or client; however this is not always feasible, as the patient or client may be too ill, language may be a problem, or a patient may be receiving medications which alter his behavior. As an alternative, an interview should be conducted with a near relative or friend. Often this is routinely done by a social worker or other intake personnel in an institution or agency; however, unless the recreation specialist has "sensitized" these personnel to the specificity of the task, information about recreation patterns and styles is usually minimal, and at times not very reliable since an awareness of the scope of possible recreation involvement requires specialized knowledge, which these other personnel do not have.

A. RECREATION PATTERNS

What is the patient's or client's current recreation pattern? In which activities does he participate alone? With others (spouse, parents, children, neighbors, friends, relatives, co-workers)? With what frequency are these participations (daily, weekly, frequently, seldom, rarely)? How intense is participation? What resources does he use for participation (home, neighborhood, special settings)? Does he belong to clubs, organizations, or special groups? Does he possess any recreation equipment of his own (camera, tape recorder, golf clubs, stamp collection, etc.)?

What was the patient's or client's past recreation pattern? (The definition of past is arbitrary, and will change in each situation. The interviewer decides upon a definition based upon the situation. For example, prior to hospitalization, prior to use of a wheelchair, prior to getting married, prior to being arrested, while still in school, etc.) What activities did he participate in? What activities did he participate in alone? With others? With what frequency were these participations? How intense were these participations? What resources did he use?

What are the future recreation plans of the patient or client? (The definition of future is also arbitrary and will depend upon the situation. For example, after discharge, when he returns home, now that he will be permanently institutionalized, when he is able to walk again, now that he will always use a wheelchair.) Are there activities he would like to engage in? Are there things he would like to learn or develop skill in? With whom would he like to do these things? What prevents him from carrying out these plans on his own?

B. RECREATION STYLE

In order to gather information about style, it is necessary to extend the "pattern questions" to elicit information of a more detailed nature. For example, if the patient or client plays golf, where does he play—on a

---

[1] Elizabeth and Karl De Schweinitz, *Interviewing in the Social Services*, London: National Council of Social Service, Publication No. 636, September 1962.

public or private golf course? If he enjoys dining out, at what type of restaurant does he usually eat—le gourmet, or a pizza parlor? If he goes to the theater or a concert, where does he usually sit? Does vacation to him mean staying home from work, camping in the woods, or a month of "air-conditioned room service by the side of a posh pool" on the Amalfi Drive? When the word "party" is used what does it conjure up in the way of place, guests, refreshments? When the word "art" is used, what does he have in mind? If he belongs to a club or an organization, what type of club is it? How involved is he in the structure and operation? How much responsibility does he take for the organization? (For additional discussion of the concept of 'style', see Chapter 8 section on 'Life Style.')

A recreation pattern indicates how one spends his time, and with whom; recreation style indicates more about the personality and character of the participant.

OBSERVATION

In order to offer adequate observational information, the patient or client should be furnished with general information about the program. Personnel would indicate that he is free to engage in those program activities which interest him. In certain situations, modifications to this procedure would be made. For example, if a patient is suicidal, he would be placed on a psychiatric service, in a nursing home if a resident is nonambulatory, in a school for the blind if a student is unfamiliar with the physical setting, in a penitentiary if maximum security rules are in effect, etc. The following are types of information the specialist can offer as the result of observation:

a. Does he come of his own volition, or does he need assistance or prodding?
b. Which activities does he choose to engage in—solitary, social, small group, aggregate, etc.?
c. With whom does he interact consistently—males, females, staff, volunteers, other patients, peers, older people, younger people, authority figures, motherly figures, no one, etc.?
d. Is he appealing to others; is he friendly, helpful, pleasant, demanding, domineering, angry, shy, noisy, quiet, pushy, etc.?

The following four cases illustrate contributions to the diagnostic and evaluation procedure;

The setting A psychiatric unit of a North American general hospital

The patient José Venedzao, male, age 12, admitted for evaluation

Social Service Report Patient is from Quatamala, son of a wealthy plantation owner. Has tried on a number of occasions to set fire to the family home. Is the oldest of three children. Has been referred by Dr. M.

to this hospital for evaluation. Family does not speak English. Mother and father have flown up with patient and have brought their own interpreter with them. Interpreter reports that patient uses "bad language" or doesn't make sense when he talks. Mother seems to be the dominant figure in the family. Father reticent to answer any questions. In discussing problem all they would indicate is that patient's language is a problem and that he tries to set fire to their house. It is my impression that they are holding back a great deal, and that the interpreter censors everything they say.

Physician's Request to Recreation Service Put the patient in a number of activities and see what you think is going on. Try to get the parents involved and find out how they react to the patient and he to each of them.

Admittedly, this is an unusual situation because of the language factor. However, it illustrates types of information that can be obtained from observation without relying upon verbal explanations. In this setting, the recreation specialist was not able to understand José, but endeavored to comply with the physician's request and contribute to the evaluation process along with nursing personnel, psychologists, social workers, and others.

With the assistance of nursing staff over a three-week period, the specialist involved José and his parents in a number of recreation activities. The following is his report to the physician:

> José is a hyperactive young man who plays hard. He doesn't seem to tire very easily. He clings to male staff on his ward during ward parties or other recreation activities, and behaves in much the same way in special activities off the ward. Sometimes he laughs with no apparent reason and there is a flood of words in Spanish, (?) during an activity. His speech seems explosive, and he appears to be angry when he speaks in this way, though there is no apparent cause for an angry outburst. He responds well to hitting and kicking games, punches a punching bag with a great deal of violence. He refuses to box with staff or other patients. He appears to be making a joke of boxing with others. José likes music, and as soon as he hears any, he begins to dance. His mother, through the interpreter, says that he likes to dance and she often dances with him at home, but he refuses to dance with her here. The dancing he does is unconventional, rather free and expressive. He engages in spontaneous solitary games such as stepping on lines in the floor pattern, jumping with both feet against the wall, and similar actions which younger children often do. In playing with a construction set, he built a rather difficult object from minimal visual instructions since he could not read the English instructions. He has constructed a jet airplane, a rocket, and a seaplane thus far. José seems to ignore his father, and although his father tries to show him how to do things, he doesn't pay any attention to him. Father doesn't seem to resent this (at least not outwardly), he just smiles at a rebuff and stands there. José won't talk with father when mother or interpreter are around to talk

to him. He addresses the interpreter in angry tones most of the time, but talks to him more than to anyone else. Very little interaction has been observed between José and his mother. She is present but doesn't try to initiate anything with him as his father tries to do. In trying to draw all three into a table tennis game, José appeared eager, but when he stood opposite his mother, he put the paddle down and left the table. Mother then said (in English!), "He is tired now, and does not wish to play." She seemed to take this as a matter of course and did not talk to him, or express any emotion, nor did she offer any further explanation. She walked away from us and just stared out of a window. José cries when left alone on the ward without his parents or the interpreter. On a few occasions he stopped crying when I brought him some picture puzzles and another construction set for use in his room. He relates positively to me and has asked the interpreter on a number of occasions to tell me that "We are friends, you and I." He also tells the interpreter to tell me other things such as, "Tell him how I was born," "I was made angry by a factory and a cow." These comments and others have to be "extracted" from the interpreter. He often refuses to repeat in English what José has said to me.

Here then is one example of the use of activity programming for diagnostic and evaluation purposes. It relies upon interaction and observation in an activity program. The following example utilizes both activity programming and interview techniques. This second example comes from an outpatient hematology clinic in a general hospital.

Medical Summary Re: Arnold Meiser, 14-year-old male, with known AHG deficiency, diagnosed at 11 months of age. Pt. has multiple hospitalizations and outpatient treatments in the past; has had multiple hemarthroses, but no deformity except for incomplete motion of the right knee joint. He had a retrobulbar hemorrhage into the right eye resulting in a degree of permanent visual loss; bleeding into the throat with tonsillitis at age 3 required a tracheotomy which is well healed. Pt. has had multiple hospital admissions because of hematuria; last episode 4 years ago revealed a left hydronephrosis with a filling defect thought to be due to a clot found on cystoscopy and retrograde phylography. Pt. is responsive to plasma or cryoprecipitate and shows no evidence of an anticoagulant.

Physician's Request to Recreation Service Social work staff is attempting to help Mrs. Meiser make future plans for Arnold. Would like impressions of pt. from recreation point of view. Note: since pt. does not attend regular school, educational input other than test scores is unavailable.

In this instance, the recreation specialist invited the patient to attend a series of activity sessions over a two-week period with other boys who came to the hospital's clinics. The patient participated in activity while his mother met with the social worker. In addition to the activity sessions, the specialist talked with the patient about his recreation involvement. The following is his report to the physician:

Arnold lives with his mother, older brother, and older sister in a private home. He awakens each weekday about 9:30 to 10:00 A.M., watches television all morning and part of the afternoon. His homestudy teacher comes about 3:00 P.M. so Arnold often doesn't do his homework until 2:00 P.M., if he does it. Teacher is there from 3 to 5 P.M. four days a week, which negates going out to play with peers who are home from school. Pt. has own room with a television set, a miniature pool table, many games and toys of his own including a camera. He goes to movies with his mother sometimes, and at other times she takes him to a private club to swim in the mornings "when it isn't crowded." Sister's boyfriend has taken him to see a football game. He used to play chess with father (deceased) and also with an uncle. Goes to church on Sundays with mother, aunt, and cousin. Cousin has encouraged him to join CYO, but mother has refused. Reports would like to play football, and would like to hunt. During activity session in the clinic he exhibits some physical limitation, particularly while standing with other boys and playing box hockey game, or shuffleboard. However, he is cheerful and stimulates involvement and interaction with the boys present. He seems to ignore physical limitations (and perhaps pain) to the best of his ability. Appears "hungry" for contact with peers in activity.

Would it be possible to change the time of the teacher's visit to the morning, so that he can become more involved in social activity outside of his home and with others than his immediate family? Is involvement in the CYO or comparable group counterindicated? Is physical therapy for conditioning purposes possible so he might develop more strength in his legs?

In this example, not only is a report provided, but the specialist has raised some questions regarding the patient's recreation pattern. In the following example of contribution to the diagnostic and evaluation process, drawn from the files of a general hospital, the patient is a 31-year-old male who has had a left leg amputation and has returned to the hospital after discharge with vague stomach complaints. An internist has requested that recreation service provide activity during the diagnostic period "as the patient tolerates." He has asked that the recreation specialist send him a report of the patient's reactions and involvement. Unlike the previous two cases, the recreation specialist is not informed how his information will be used. After eighteen days, this is an excerpt of the specialist's report:

Mr. Taniant is a rather surly individual who sneers at the program and the staff. Although he attempts to socialize somewhat with other patients, he has developed no regular relationships with any specific person. His attendance is erratic, and he blames this on his "pain." He repeatedly says that he should be getting medication for his "stomach ulcer" and that he isn't being treated correctly. He expresses a great deal of hostility toward the medical staff and toward the hospital in general. When he has been invited to join in an activity by staff or patients, he responds that he can't because of his prosthesis. He indicates that he is not as adequate as he was before he lost his leg. He has mentioned on a number of occasions that he was not really sure he had to lose his leg. At other times he derides himself, and there is a considerable degree of self-belittling.

The last example of this element of service is from the files of a large metropolitan general hospital homecare clinic. The recreation specialist was asked to interview the client in her home and report the findings of the interview to the homecare team.

Mrs. T. Z., age 71, lives alone, 2-room flat, elevator building, public housing project. Arteriosclerotic heart disease; functional classification IIC; histamine type allergy to some foods and drugs; hypotension; mild emphysema; fibrosis; partial gastric resection with gastrojejunostomy cholecystectomy; mild cardiac, cirrhosis of liver.

On homecare since April, expected to remain indefinitely. Ambulatory and independent in activities of daily living. Homecare service provides housekeeper three days a week to clean and shop. Prior to illness, describes self as a "very active woman." Worked full time, active in churchwork, did a great deal of sewing and crocheting.

Now spends most of time listening to the radio, watching television. Reads Bible, religious magazines, newspapers regularly, exchanges visits with neighbors fairly frequently. Goes to a nearby church most Sundays; on special occasions takes taxi to own church, which is too far to walk to. On Thursday afternoons, when feeling well enough, attends golden age club which meets once a week in her housing project. Expressed desire to have this facility opened more frequently. Would like to attend Eastview Center, but can no longer get there; it is too far for her to walk to, and is not convenient to public transportation, nor can she afford regular taxi fare. Expressed a desire to get out of the house more often, learn how to knit, and have opportunities to learn some of the handcrafts taught at the senior citizens' centers. Stated that she would get out more if she lived on a lower floor, but is afraid of being stuck in elevators.

In the first and third reports, observation was the major technique in gathering information, while in the second and fourth cases, interview was used. Dependent upon the knowledge and experience of the recreation specialist, information may be called for in a summary report and used to augment other information in the diagnostic or evaluation process. It may be presented by the specialist in a case conference at which time the specialist might be asked to render an opinion or judgment or interpret his findings in light of the other information being presented. The specialist may be told how his information will be used, or he may not know this. In some situations his contribution may be quite important to the process, while in other instances it may be peripheral.

Elements of Service: Part II 89

Programming For Treatment Purposes And In Care-Plans

With respect to activity programming for treatment purposes, it must be remembered that recreative experience is a "nonspecific" in regard to pathology, and must not be construed as therapy per se (See Chapter 3, p. 19). However, it is possible in certain circumstances to contribute to the active treatment program designed for a patient or client in very specific ways. The value of recreation in the treatment of children has had international recognition for a number of years.[2] Its use for this purpose with adults is less well documented.

The therapeutic recreation specialist can use himself as a "therapeutic agent," or he can use aspects of the program itself as part of the treatment regime. The following are some typical requests for recreation service that indicate direct contribution to a treatment process in a general hospital and in a psychiatric hospital.

GENERAL HOSPITAL

Post-operative; left temporal lobe ablation; patient is withdrawn and afraid of seizures; eats compulsively; help patient to regain self-confidence and animation, help him to socialize.

Post-operative; pituitary tumor; progressive visual loss; patient receiving therapeutic X-ray; assist the patient in adjustment to his disability.

Plastic surgery; industrial accident, both legs grafted; patient will be in a wheelchair for minimum of 2 months, was active in sports and weight-lifting; attempt to relieve psychic tension and prevent depression.

Post-operative; right hip pinned; no weight-bearing; help patient socialize and maintain outgoing capacity and skills.

Fractured back; body cast, bed-bound for undetermined period; can use hands well; divert attention from pain and discomfort, make stay tolerable.

Neurodermatitis; help patient adjust to routine and expend energy. Do not let patient engage in activity that will cause him to perspire.

PSYCHIATRIC HOSPITAL

Agitated depression; suicidal; firm, positive, encouraging approach; allow time for ruminations and self-recriminations during activity; use activity to ventilate aggressive feelings.

[2] "Play—The Sick Child's Lifeline," *World Medicine*, January 4, 1966, pp. 23-31; Grace Langdon, "A Study of the Uses of Toys in a Hospital," *Child Development*, XIX, No. 4 (December 1948), 197-212.

Acute anxiety reaction; shy with females, timid; increase self-esteem, strengthen masculine image and feelings.

Conversion reaction; epilepsy; passive dependent personality; help build self-confidence.

Organic brain involvement; encephalitis; patient aware of condition; needs encouragement and praise; may be able to return to work as tool designer eventually; strengthen socialization.

Chronic brain syndrome; undetermined nature; reacts in a dependent and hostile manner; no plan for the future; encourage self-sufficiency and self-expression.

In each of these orders, the request deals with factors that influence the total treatment of the patient. The recreation specialist does not deal with the primary pathological problem as do other members of the treatment team, but rather he is asked to concern himself with the social and emotional aspects of the patient's life—aspects that bear upon the primary problem. In some instances the specialist can use recreation activity to comply with an order, while at other times it is how the specialist uses himself in relation to the patient that is important. Both of these aspects of practice will be discussed in more detail in subsequent chapters of this section.

To illustrate how a recreation specialist might comply with a treatment order, excerpts from a long case record are presented.

Rx RECREATION

Establish accepting relationship with patient. Allow him to involve himself at his own rate of speed. Initially provide for individual activity, but gradually move the patient toward more social experience. Permit self-recrimination. Report progress weekly.

PROGRESS REPORTS (SUMMARIZED)

Arthur Smith, male white, age 32, married, two children. Admitted 3/10. Family hospitalized patient because of suicide attempt. Patient is socially prominent dentist who was being blackmailed for involving himself sexually with a patient in his office. Referred to the Recreation Department on 3/20. Patient came for initial interview to recreation specialist's office. He was soft-spoken, rather pleasant-looking, appeared somewhat anxious. He talked about doing some tape-recorded plays in order to practice acting. He said he had always wanted to act. A time was agreed upon for daily activity. He appeared for the first session on the following day, did not interact at all with the other patients involved in the activity, stood on the fringes throughout the session, and left midway into the session without a word to anyone. He did not come back on the second day, nor did he return throughout the week.

The specialist went to see him on 3/27. Found him reading in the dayroom on his ward. Sat next to him and asked why he didn't come back. He said he wasn't ready to be with other people, and wanted to do something alone. The specialist offered him a number of other activities, and he selected music listening. He came to the music room that afternoon, and with the help of the specialist he selected recordings for an hour of listening by himself. He selected mournful, sad, morose music.

On 4/1, the specialist asked if he would mind if another patient or two listened to the music with him. He agreed to this request.

Third week of activity: Smith came to the specialist and asked some questions about becoming an actor. He said, "... I can't really do this though, because I'm a married man with children." Each day he kept talking about the play-reading group and said he was going to come back to it, but he kept putting this off.

Fourth week—the specialist said that he could join the play-reading group at any time, and not to feel pressured. Smith responded that he "expected to be hospitalized a long time, and would have the opportunity to do many things in the recreation department."

Fifth week—staff noted some behavioral change in Smith. He asked that he be called "Arty" by staff. He began to show up at many recreation activities and introduced himself to staff, patients, and volunteers as "Sam Schultz," "Joe Green," and "A. Nonymous." He did clever verbal characterizations of a humorous nature which were appropriate to the name he had taken. No one questioned who he really was, and realizing he was joking, praised him accordingly.

Seventh week—Smith now states that he wants to sell his practice and talks to the recreation specialist about becoming a college teacher of zoology. He avoids talking about his private life with other patients, and will only enter into conversations about the activity or nondescript subjects. Yesterday he took his first piano lesson, and continues to be active with the play-reading group. He shows up at evening social functions, and has moved from the status of isolate to that of leader in many activities.

By contrast, the following illustration indicates how the therapeutic recreation specialist contributes directly to the treatment plan for a patient who has a physical disorder. The setting is a typical general hospital.

The Patient: John J. Tribuen, 26 years old, male, married, no children, admitted 7/14

Diagnosis: pleural effusion (TBC)

Social History: Pt. is of Italian decent, from a large family, laboring class. Pt. has some college education and is employed as a salesman for an asphalt firm. Travels a good deal. Wife unavailable for interview. Pt.'s mother states wife is not "kind" to her son, since he is in hospital and wife has decided to go visit a friend in New Orleans. Pt. is Catholic, wife is not. Mother gives the impression that daughter-in-law is not a "good woman." Pt. married for four months. Met wife at a dance.

The situation may be one of a hasty marriage and now an estrangement, or just sour grapes on the part of the mother. Not enough material to go on, since wife is unavailable for interview.

Physician's Order for Recreation Service: Above-named patient will be confined to bed and room for approximately six months. Because of emotional factors that co-exist in this situation, request the following: (1) encourage patient to cooperate with ward procedures; (2) relieve tension and anxiety; (3) gradually increase activity tolerance. (Note: do not physically tire the patient during the first few weeks. We want him to stay in bed, with as little exertion as possible until the effusion has subsided.) Record progress notes on chart.

Recreation Progress Notes 7/19–Preliminary interview reveals pt. has some interest in photography and reading (appropriate activity for physical limitations), pt. appears angry, belligerent, and quite restless. Discussed activity plan with him.

7/27–Provided pt. with a selection of books from the library, and developed plans to take photographs in room, still life, etc. Also used rear-view projector to show pt. a film on photography techniques. Pt. appears less belligerent, but is still quite restless. Seems to be becoming depressed.

7/31–Pt. said he had to talk with someone. Couldn't stand the SW who kept bothering him, and anyway, women were all "pigs." Pt. wanted to see a priest. Pt. began crying and explained he had a letter from his wife. He said that she "was whoring all over New Orleans." Said, what good was he in the hospital for so long. Asked what about later when he got out? Calmed him down, and promised to send for the priest. Listened to him, but did not offer advice, except to indicate that SW may be able to help, and probably had a contact in New Orleans. Pt. said he felt better, now that he had talked to someone about it. Said I probably thought that he was an "ass," but he loved his wife. I reassured him that in his situation things do get difficult, and would not think the less of him for the outburst. I promised to see him again at the regular time next week.

Note to Dr. H. It is becoming more apparent that we cannot continue to comply with your request, unless some additional help is forthcoming in relation to Mr. T's emotional status.

10/4–Pt. in process of planning his "one-man" photo show for the lounge, as soon as permission is given him to leave his room. His extension course studies are progressing well, and pt. plans to return to college. He does not talk much about his wife or his home situation any more, and the little he does mention concerns the status quo. He has mentioned that he has made a "mistake," but I have tried to reassure him regarding his ability to face the future. Will begin planning to introduce new activity schedule for him as soon as he is permitted to leave his room and use the other facilities.

Programming for treatment purposes usually concerns an acute condition and a short-term goal. On the other hand, a "care plan" is a term often used to describe the total treatment a patient or client receives in a long-term setting such as a nursing home or continued treatment center. In a school for the mentally retarded or a school for the blind, the term might be "educational plan," while in a correction setting it might be referred to as a "rehabilitation plan." The following notes from a "Care Planning Review Conference" in a long-term care setting illustrates this aspect of service.

Miss L. T., age 87, advanced cataract condition, eyesight very poor, ambulatory, hearing good. Resident has been in the setting for four years. Complains about her roommate. Reports that her roommate plays her television set too loudly, will only allow a small lamp to be lit in the room, and has visitors frequently who "take over the room." Indicates that she is not getting enough "mental stimulation."

Nursing staff reports that resident has difficulty ambulating by herself. Seems to function adequately and cares for self with minimal assistance. Social Service reports resident has few visitors, seems to be more depressed since being moved to current room two months ago after last CPR conference. Medical report indicates that resident is in good health except for visual condition, is alert, and no medical risk at this time.

Recreation reports that resident is active in recreation program, spends time with music listening group, attends theater excursions out of the Center, and is quite social—visiting other residents who are less ambulant. Resident appears alert, optimistic, and interested.

Action: Social Service will attempt to determine why she has few visitors. Nursing will arrange transfer to different room as soon as feasible. Recreation will explore resident involvement in weekly discussion group.

The following excerpt illustrates similar aspects of recreation programming in a correctional setting. The material regards a second offender.

L. L., age 17, progress report for planning purposes: This is his second try with us, and quite different from the first. During his first "go-round" he was uncooperative and difficult to get along with. This is no longer the case. He appears more passive and easygoing. He is getting along well with peers, and is taking an active part in many recreation activities. He is demonstrating some leadership capacity by coordinating a sports "smoker" twice a week. He appears to be pleasant and dependable at this time. This all is in marked contrast to his former behavior, which put him into conflict with staff members and certain peers who are "authority" figures. He wouldn't give up on trying to "see what he could get away with." This type of behavior is not evident at present. He obeys all rules. He has also begun to express some positive comments about his situation here. This change from an aggressively hostile person to a pleasant cooperative person is inconsistent, and may not be reliable.

Programming for Altered Life Situations

Sometimes, and particularly with regard to severe physical disability, treatment will alter a person's life situation. That is, he will no longer be able to live in the way that he did prior to treatment. The advent of an amputation, the application of a prosthesis, acute loss of vision or hearing, inability to walk or use a hand—all of these require that a person learn to make optimal use of himself in a different way. It has been reported that persons who are subject to this type of alteration in their life situation seem to follow a similar emotional pattern. First they mourn the loss of the capacity or ability and behave in a brooding or bereaved fashion, much as one would with the death of a loved one. A second stage is marked by bewilderment, sometimes agitated and depressed feelings, and often increased dependence. In some instances there is also belligerence. The third stage finds the person alert, responsible, and eager to learn and develop existing capacities and abilities to compensate for the loss.

During the first stage, a number of treatment personnel play an active part in the care process. Recreation's role is minimal and might be primarily entertaining. During the second stage, recreation activity may be offered to permit ventilation of angry feelings and to strengthen feelings of self-worth and independence. In the event that the second state becomes elongated, direct psychiatric intervention may be required. In the third stage, recreation and vocational services have a major role to play. It is during this period that the person is offered a range of opportunities which will allow him to explore recreation experiences in which he will meet with a high degree of success and personal satisfaction through the development of new skills and the use of dormant capacities and abilities.

The following case material from a rehabilitation unit in a hospital illustrates this element of service.

> Mr. R. Shasky, age 42, single: automobile accident. Patient will be confined to wheelchair for a time, and will eventually be fitted with a leg brace.
>
> **Summary Report from Recreation Department**: Mr. Shasky has been invited to attend a number of recreation activities over the past eight weeks. He required assistance with his wheelchair at movies, shows, etc., indicating that he was afraid and refused to move the chair by himself. He is a pinochle player, and for the first few times he was wheeled to a table with others, but now does this himself. He relates well to other patients

during activity sessions, and has established a positive relationship with the recreation staff. He appears to have some difficulty in accepting help from others, as when volunteers offer him assistance at a refreshment table, he will refuse coffee, etc., unless he can take it himself. He expresses some anxiety about his condition, and when recreation staff suggests some other aspects of program in which he could become involved, he declines, indicating that he is inadequate.

During one of the evening activities, his sister was visiting and came to the program with him. Mr. Shasky was particularly anxious and dependent then. Sister appeared to be rather aggressive and forward. She bullied and disparaged Mr. Shasky a great deal during the evening, and would not let him do as he wished.

Fifth-Month Summary Report from Recreation Department: Mr. Shasky is becoming quite active in a variety of activities and asserting his independence. However, during last week of this period a great deal of regression was noted.

On Monday, Mr. Shasky told the recreation specialist that he would be leaving the hospital shortly, probably by the end of the week. He talked at great length about all the things that he would still like to do in the program. He said he didn't want to leave the hospital, except that his sister kept reminding him that he was perfectly able to live at home and come back to the clinic for treatment, and that he was taking up a bed from someone who could use it more than he. He spent some time in the hobby shop finishing up a project, and then he returned to his room.

On Tuesday, he came into the game lounge for a few minutes before the other patients arrived, and again talked to the specialist about his situation, but with less enthusiasm and more anxiety. During his pinochle game he told the other players that he couldn't concentrate (very unlike him) and that he wanted to stop playing. He told them that he really didn't understand why he should leave, since he was still sick, but obviously, "the doctor knows best." He asked to be helped back to his room, something he has not done for many weeks.

Special Report From Recreation Department: On Wednesday, Mr. Shasky came to the recreation specialist's office to say he wouldn't participate in any activities today—in fact, he wasn't going to physical therapy clinic either. He again brought up his future situation and his concerns. It was suggested that he talk with the SW about them. He replied that he wanted as little to do with the SW as possible. He said it was easier for him to talk to a man, or someone who "really" understands. Note to Social Service: Is discharge a medical decision? Was patient involved in decision process? How much is sister involved?

On Friday, Mr. Shasky came to the game lounge at the usual time with a large grin on his face and announced that his brace was bent and there was some pain in his leg and that he would not be discharged. He told the other patients that his doctor felt that he should stay until he was "really" well enough to be discharged. He was quite relaxed, less tense, and very much at ease. He spent most of the afternoon in the lounge. At one point, he offered to go to the canteen to bring back coffee for himself and the other players at his table. When one player suggested that it would be too difficult for him, he replied that it would be easy and he could do it.

Seventh-Month Summary Report from Recreation Department: Mr. Shasky has been exposed to a variety of community activities during this period. He seems to appreciate trips to horse races, and declines the theater. He is able to ambulate quite well with his brace and cane, demonstrating his ability to other patients at a cafeteria in town yesterday. He indicates that he used to be "quite a dancer" but recognizes that is no longer feasible. We have given him an opportunity to try fly casting in lieu of other sports he used to engage in. Lately, he has begun to talk about leaving the hospital and getting out and "making some money," so he can "really" enjoy himself. He has told his pinochle buddies that the vocational counselor is very helpful, and that they were making some vocational plans for his future.

Programming as an Aspect of Predischarge Counseling

This area of activity programming has been documented for a considerable number of years.[3] At first, programming for this purpose could be found only in large publicly owned psychiatric institutions, but later similar service was found in rehabilitation settings of various types. In a study[4] of approximately 300 institutions in the United States which offer therapeutic recreation service, a little over 50 percent report predischarge and counseling activity as part of the recreation service. The intent of this element of service is to enable the patient or client to examine the recreation aspect of his life before he leaves the institution and to see this in relation to the other aspects of his existence. There is no specific method of selecting patients or clients for this service—this depends upon their situation and the judgment of the total staff in an institution who are responsible for predischarge planning or institutional release. With respect to the recreation aspect of the process, both individual and group techniques are employed. Individual sessions may be conducted by a therapeutic recreation specialist, a psychologist, a social worker, or a nurse, while group sessions usually involve a recreation specialist and one or more of the other personnel. In some instances group sessions involve resource persons, such as recreation personnel from the community. Group discussion sessions are usually held for an hour

---

[3] See W. I. Olson and J. B. McCormic, "Recreation Counseling in the Psychiatric Service of a General Hospital," *Journal of Nervous and Mental Disease*, CXXV (April-June 1957), 237-39; S. H. Acuff, "Recreation Counseling as an Aspect of Programming for the Short-Term Psychiatric Patient," *Recreation in Treatment Centers*, V (September 1966) 5-7; F. B. Arje, "Recreation Counseling," *Hospital Management*, LXXXIX (April 1960), 2-3.

[4] G. S. O'Morrow, *A Study of Recreation Service to Psychiatric Patients in Relation to Pre-Discharge Planning and Aftercare*, (New York: Teachers College, Columbia University, unpublished doctoral dissertation, 1969).

once a week over a variable period of two or more months, while individual sessions during this period may vary from half an hour to an hour.

Simultaneous to individual or group discussion sessions, specific activity sessions are usually offered to permit the patient or client to explore a range of interests. These activities are designed to provide a nonsheltered experience. Often, many of these sessions are conducted outside of the institution, utilizing regular community recreation resources. This latter aspect not only provides a more diversified and realistic approach for the patient or client, but it also familiarizes him with what the community has to offer. Generally, predischarge counseling activity is offered with a variety of objectives in mind, namely:

—To enable patients and clients to strengthen existing social ties with individuals and groups, and to form new social ties;
—To enable patients and clients to understand how to identify, locate, and use recreation resources; and
—To enable patients and clients to recognize the meaning of recreation in their lives.

During counseling sessions, attitudes toward recreation are explored; recreation needs as they relate to age, education, family, socioeconomic, and cultural status are discussed; and information concerning community recreation resources is provided. In some instances, direct referral to community recreation agencies is made to assist the patient or client to make contact after discharge. This may include a single telephone call to a colleague in a community recreation setting by the therapeutic recreation specialist, or a simple letter of introduction. It may amount to a more formal social agency referral procedure. In addition to trips to spectator athletic events, theaters, and a variety of social events, some institutions offer opportunities to engage in activities of a service nature, such as volunteering in community agencies.

As a concomitant of this type of service, some institutions have found it necessary to extend the service after discharge, and a number of patterns can be identified for this purpose. Some institutions form a special club for discharged patients or clients who then return to the institution for activity and further counseling sessions once a week. Some communities have established transitional social programs for this purpose, and dischargees are referred to these programs on a formal basis when they are not ready to recreate on their own. This "halfway" measure provides for a person to live and work in the community but to continue to use the laboratory approach to recreation for a time.[5]

---

[5] See Mabel Palmer, *The Social Club* (New York: National Association for Mental Health, 1966); Joshua Bieren, "Great Britain's Therapeutic Social Clubs," *Mental Hospitals,* XII, No. 4 (April 1962) 203-207; National Institute of Mental Health, *Community Care of the Mentally Ill: A Selected Annotated Bibliography,* Chapter IV; "After-Care Facilities," U.S. Public Health Publication No. 1527, Bibliography Series No. 69, 1966; R. S. Felixson, *Leisure Services and Mental Health Rehabilitation* (Los Angeles: Recreation and Youth Service Planning Council, 1965).

These special programs may be offered by a municipal recreation department, a YWCA, or a separate agency such as Fountain House in New York, Circle F Club in Minneapolis, Horizon House in Philadelphia, and Fellowship Club in San Francisco. Some of these programs cater to persons who have been mentally ill, while others are primarily concerned with former addicts. There are certain similar community programs for mentally retarded adolescents and young adults, some for parolees from correctional institutions, and certain combined vocational and recreational programs for the physically disabled person who is in transition from a rehabilitation setting. These "halfway" programs are not to be confused with "sheltered" programs, which are discussed in the next section of this chapter. "Halfway" programs are transitional and it is assumed that participants will not need the support that they offer after a short period of time. When more than transitional recreation service is required, a community may offer a variety of residential programs such as Day Hospitals, Night Hospitals, Weekend Hospitals, Halfway Houses, and other flexible community residential agencies. These programs provide residential care as well as recreation service while the resident is employed in the community in a regular occupation or is training for employment. Many of these programs have become necessary throughout the world, because residential psychiatric facilities have for the most part been built away from urban centers and sources of employment.[6]

The following excerpt from a case record in a rehabilitation center illustrates an individual predischarge counseling session.

> Mr. H. Steel, Age 28, married, 2 children, quadriplegia polio residuals; (4th session)
>
> Again in this session Mr. Steel talked about his disappointment regarding a career in hospital administration. He reiterated how long he had planned for this career and his intention regarding graduate study. We went over the same ground regarding the refusal of the University to accept him because of his degree of disability, and he showed me a letter from another university indicating the same information, "inasmuch as the task of an administrator makes a great many physical demands upon the incumbent, we are sorry to say . . ." He indicated that since this was the third letter of this type, he'd better get used to the idea of doing something else. He said he had been discussing this with Mr. Nattano, his social worker, as well as discussing his housing problems.
>
> We then talked about some of his recreation interests, and he led into a discussion of activity with his wife and children. He expressed concern and doubt about his ability to maintain a social life with his wife, and questioned how much of a father he could really be to his children. He said that it would be easier to stay in bed and read a book than try to

---

[6] See David Landy and Milton Greenblatt, *Halfway House* (Washington, D.C.: U.S. Gov't Printing Office, 1969); B. M. Kramer, *Day Hospital* (New York: Frune & Stratton, 1962).

attend social activities. We spent some time exploring types of activities he might engage in with his wife which could be shared in spite of his physical limitations. We decided to invite his wife to join some of the predischarge group activities with him, and attempt to test out kinds of things which they both might enjoy. He recognized that he might have to learn some new skills, and that his wife might have to assist him in this endeavor. We did some planning regarding a series of trips to town with other married couples in the group who are faced with similar problems. I indicated this would help him identify exactly what would be involved. He understood from the discussion that he must try and function as a normal social individual within the framework of his limitations rather than retreating from sociability.

We decided to talk at our next session about the father-children situation. I reassured him that there were a number of activities which they would like and in which he might engage them. I promised to bring some material for him to read about these activities.

The following edited excerpt from a recreation department report of a special activity session in a psychiatric hospital illustrates a group session that is part of the predischarge activity process. The group includes Mr. B., the recreation specialist, Miss N., a nurse, and two volunteers, Mr. and Mrs. K., as staff, and five patients. Three of the patients are married and their spouses have been invited to join the group. The patients are Mr. T., Mr. H., Mrs. R., Mr. M., and Mr. L. The spouses are Mrs. T., Mrs. H., and Mr. R. The activity is a spaghetti dinner at a local community restaurant, the Casa Salerno, and then seats at the Ice Show at the municipal arena.

Dinner was organized as two separate groups at two tables: Miss N., Mr. and Mrs. K., Mr. and Mrs. T., and Mr. M. in one group, and Mr. L., Mr. and Mrs. H., Mr. and Mrs. R., and myself in the second group. Miss N. drove one car and I drove the other. At the Ice Show, Mrs. K. sat with group two, and Mr. L. sat with group one. After the Ice Show we had coffee at the Pancake House and discussed the evening.

The patients in group two indicated that at times they were at a loss for "small talk" at the dinner table, and Mr. T. said he felt this way also, but watched Mr. and Mrs. K. (the volunteers) and got some clues from them. We then spent some time on "small talk." Mrs. R. said the crowd at the arena troubled her, but something Mrs. K. said made her realize that others have the same feelings, and so she felt she could handle it. Mr. L. indicated that he wished we had better seats, and that led to a discussion of costs and budgeting for recreation activities such as this type of evening out. Mrs. H. said she wanted to thank the staff because she really enjoyed the evening. She said Mr. H. never took her to an ice show before. Mr. H. responded that he didn't think she'd like anything like that. Mrs. H. then said, "You never asked me if I would." We then discussed the mechanics of planning for an evening out. Mr. and Mrs. K. told how they do it, indicating that either may take the initiative, but they discussed it before making a definite commitment for the other. Mr. L. said he used to argue with his fiancée about what they would do, and he always let her have her way. He said this was before his hospitalization, and things will be different now, since he knows this is not the thing to do. He said that he was looking for a different kind of girl now. I indicated that it was time to go. The five patients returned to the hospital with me. Miss N. took the others.

Programming for Sheltered Experience

This element of service is usually operable in special settings administered by health agencies, social agencies, or public recreation departments. Service is geared to persons who have disorders that preclude their use of usual recreation resources in the community. This element of service may be viewed as a goal-oriented continuum which aims at enabling participants to reach their highest possible level of social independence. With this long-range goal in view, the continuum provides for five levels of programming. Depending on the individual participant's degree of limitation, each level can be regarded either as a step to the next level or as the optimum level of performance in social and recreative activity that can be expected for a given participant.

Usually service is provided in a nonresidential setting, but one or more levels of the continuum may be operant in a long-term care setting. No single community agency may provide all five levels of programming, but rather service may be offered in a coordinated fashion within one locality by a group of agencies.

This continuum includes the following five levels of programmming:

Programming for the isolated person
Programming for the secluded person
Programming for the limited person
Programming for the included person
Programming for the independent person

THE ISOLATED PERSON

Persons needing this level of programming are usually ill or disabled children or adults who have had little or no opportunity to be with others outside their homes. Recreation personnel, trained volunteers, and parents or surrogates work together to help the individual within the home setting explore and experiment with activities that promote development of: (a) psychophysical skills; and (b) a concept of mastery over inanimate objects. Equipment is made available through a number of sources—the public library, a recreation agency, a social agency—or is purchased outright. When a participant expresses interest in learning a particular activity skill, personnel with special leadership skills go into the home to teach the skill to the participant and his family. Activities are encouraged that provide immediate satisfaction for the individual, as well as activities that promote healthful interaction and participation among all those who are part of the home situation.

When feasible, activities involving minimal social interaction with peers are arranged in and outside of the home; for example, correspondence and telephone conversations with peers in special programs, followed by brief visits to these programs for a special event. As the participant acquires new recreative skills, interpersonal as well as activity skills, the latter may serve to prepare him for participation with peers in the next level of programming.

It is apparent that logistical problems may make taking the "isolated" person out of the home an impossible task, such as living in a high-rise nonelevator building, or not having access to adequate transportation. However, this limitation does not prevent the use of the other techniques, nor of having others in for a visit.[7]

THE SECLUDED PERSON

Ill or disabled children and adults who have had some opportunities to acquire recreation knowledge, skill, and experience may be served at an ordinary community facility if their limitations permit their attendance. Personnel in this facility are professionally prepared to establish special groups for disabled persons with respect to chronological age and degree of disability, as well as level of recreative skill. Programming is intended to: (a) develop further skills, (b) expand social interaction experiences, (c) offer appropriate activities wifh respect to age; for example, prevocational opportunities for the older teenager or young adult, community service activity for the older participant. When an individual shows readiness and has developed a number of interpersonal as well as recreation skills and abilities, he is gradually introduced to aggregate activity with some nondisabled persons who attend other recreation programs within the facility. This latter experience may serve to prepare the participant for involvement in the next level of programming.[8]

Some programs for the secluded person serve the same members for many years. These persons, because of limitations imposed by their disability, cannot achieve the degree of social independence and skill necessary for interaction in more advanced programs. However, caution must be taken to avoid the possibility that a person may be "stuck" in this type of program. It is

[7] M. D. McMullin, *How to Help the Shut-In Child* (New York: E. P. Dutton and Co., Inc., 1954); M. K. Rich, *Handcrafts for the Homebound* (Springfield Ill.: Charles C. Thomas, Inc., 1960).

[8] Arthur Schwartz, *Social and Recreation Patterns of Orthopedically Handicapped Children* (New York: Associated YM-YWHA, 1962), Project on Camp and City Leisure Time Services, *First the Person, Then the Disability* (Chicago: Metropolitan Welfare Council, n.d.); Irving Miller, *Recreation Services for Deaf-Blind Persons* (New York: Industrial Home For The Blind, 1959).

extremely important to establish groups with respect to chronological age, and to program realistically with respect to age. For example, if a 12-year-old mentally retarded boy is in a "secluded" program, he should be placed in a group for preteenagers, not in a group with preschoolers or in a group with adults. The activities in which his group engages should be appropriate for preteens. Even in instances in which preteenagers do not develop the kinds of skills required for successful participation at another level of performance as they become chronologically older, they should be exposed to activities appropriate to chronological age and physical maturation level. It has become apparent in the past few years that the mass media influences psychic maturation to some degree; one should not expect persons who are aware of astronauts and their trips to the moon to sit coloring paper plates or stringing large colored beads. On the contrary, programming must be meaningful and realistic with regard to the world about them, for they are not "secluded" 24 hours a day, all week long.

THE LIMITED PERSON

For disabled children and adults who have successful recreative experiences with a few nondisabled peers and have been able to use at least one neighborhood recreation resource, opportunities should be provided to enable them to join ongoing interest groups and clubs available to nondisabled persons within their own neighborhood recreation centers. Gradually they should be helped to increase their range of social interaction, developing greater social independence and skill in using additional neighborhood recreation resources. In some instances, participants in this type of program may need to remain for some time in a small group, but for many activities they may be capable of joining large groups of nondisabled persons. Successful progression toward independent participation of this kind depends on the limitations imposed by disability and the quality of leadership service. In addition to leadership, persons in this level of programming may need some advice and counseling assistance to work through anxieties. On the average, many persons with disability can engage in a program for "limited" persons. There will be some activities that they can successfully engage in with nondisabled peers, and others in which they continue to need "sheltered" situations. A person who is confined to a wheelchair, for example, will always have some difficulty engaging in activities that require traveling, such as trips to the theater; however, this same person's limitations need not affect his participation in a choral group that has its practice sessions at a neighborhood community center or church and performs in the same facility. In this level of program it must be remembered that the "limited" person is not totally limited in all areas of recreation, regardless of his disability.[9]

[9] "What About the Handicapped Child In the Group?" *Potentials*, New York Service for the Orthopedically Handicapped, II, No. 1 (May 1967).

Elements of Service: Part II 103

THE INCLUDED PERSON

In programs serving limited persons who are able to use some of the recreation resources of their home neighborhood, arrangements can be made for them to have opportunities for expanded social interaction with nondisabled persons. The use of neighborhood program directories, newsletters, local newspapers, and the like would be a vehicle for informing disabled persons of activities that are going on in the neighborhood. Organized clubs, church groups, and others would be asked to keep disabled persons informed of activities open to the public so that all may be "included." The intent is to engage in a broader range of activities in this level of program so that one may prepare for successful participation at the next level.

THE INDEPENDENT PERSON

When there is successful interaction with many nondisabled peers in one's own neighborhood, recreation personnel can provide information and referral to facilitate broader use of recreation resources such as beaches, pools, zoos, museums, concerts, camps, restaurants, special events, and the like. In programming for the "independent" person, emphasis is placed upon providing public information and education to encourage nondisabled persons to make community recreation resources more accessible to persons with disability. Counseling the disabled person's family and friends is often necessary to indicate how they can participate in a wide variety of activities with the participant. The intent in this level of programming is to enable the disabled person to act independently and no longer need specialized programs; however, such resources as modified transportation, unique directories, and altered equipment may be necessary for him to function independently.[10]

The material in this chapter concerns the concept of activity programming in therapeutic recreation service. Little has been said about the organization and structure of program. Much of the literature in the total field of recreation concerns some aspects of programming. The following chapters offer a brief review of programming concepts as they apply to therapeutic recreation service.

---

[10] K. E. Evans, *Sport and Physical Recreation for the Disabled* (London: Disabled Living Foundation, 1970).

III
SOCIAL AND BEHAVIORAL FACTORS IN PROGRAMMING

In the field of recreation, the word "program" means more than just a listing of activities that are offered to potential participants. Program is the matrix of service offered by the recreation staff. It alludes to a cohesive plan that takes into account the interaction of a variety of factors.

This section examines many of these factors in considerable detail with regard to certain knowledges from the behavioral and social sciences. Program is viewed first from the point of view of "development" or the "process of planning." Application of social science information to the development of program is offered in Chapter 8. In addition, an application of systems analysis procedures in therapeutic recreation program planning is presented in Chapter 9. This latter material will be of special interest to personnel in larger, more sophisticated settings that use systems procedures. It also offers the researcher a way of structuring evaluative research.

The second part of the section examines program organization in light of social and behavior science—principally sociology and social psychology. Aspects of applicable group dynamics information is also included in this chapter. Program content is looked at with respect to the participant and the behavioral domains.

The final chapter of the section offers a range of case material and questions for application of material presented in the text. It offers stimulus for continued dialogue and discussion.

8
Social and Behavioral Factors in Program Development

Most recreation program planning in the past has been based upon lists of principles. These lists, while promulgating a range of positive social values, are nonsystematic and do not lend themselves to specific procedures that result in definitive and measurable outcomes. For example, when examining a number of contemporary recreation texts,[1] all principles and guidelines seem to start with the phrase "program should..." or "program must..." and then include some or all of the following:

—Be developed to meet important needs
—Be planned realistically with regard to participants
—Be efficient
—Consider existing services and potential resources
—Have diversity and balance
—Involve challenge
—Insure maximum participation
—Possess adequate financial support

[1] See R. E. Carlson, T. R. Deppe, and J. R. Maclean, *Recreation in American Life* (Belmont, California: Wordsworth Publishing Co., Inc., 1967), pp. 357-78; H. G. Danford, *Creative Leadership in Recreation* (Boston: Allyn and Bacon, 1964), pp. 122-34; V. Frye and M. Peters, *Therapeutic Recreation* (Harrisburg, Pa.: Stackpole Books, 1972), pp. 165-66; R. G. Kraus, *Recreation Today: Program Planning and Leadership* (New York: Appleton-Century-Crofts, 1966), pp. 249-53; H. D. Meyer and C. K. Brightbill, *Recreation Administration* (Englewood Cliffs, N.J.: Prentice-Hall, Inc., 1956), pp. 345-52, J. Pomeroy, *Recreation for the Physically Handicapped* (New York: The Macmillan Co., 1964), pp. 71-74; L. S. Rodney, *Administration of Public Recreation* (New York: The Ronald Press, 1964), pp. 204-206.

Social and Behavioral Factors in Program Development

—Include thoughtful evaluations
—Demonstrate imaginative use of resources
—Use qualified leadership and supervision

There is no value in arguing the merit or lack of merit in this approach to programming; however, it is important to note that advances in the social and behavioral sciences insure that planning no longer need be undertaken with only a "set of good intentions." One may now proceed on a more organized and systematic basis when engaging in program planning by using findings of these sciences.

In order to adequately develop a cohesive program plan, certain social variables that influence a potential participant's perception of a program must be acknowledged. Some of these follow.

SANCTION

Because an activity is included in a program, it implies that an authority figure in the administrative hierarchy of the institution or agency has approved the activity. In effect, he has said, "It is alright to engage in this activity. You have approval." To some patients and clients, sanction to participate is of paramount importance and must take the form of a verbal invitation from a staff member or appear on a printed listing of activities.

LEADERSHIP

This factor indicates that consideration has been given to scheduling and budgeting of staff time with regard to other staff responsibilities. It implies that direct supervision of patient or client behavior is available. This may be of prime importance to some potential participants, as well as to members of the institutional or agency staff. It extends the concept of sanction by assuring the physical presence of personnel. It also implies that thoughtful consideration has been given to the nature of required leadership for a given activity, and offers a sense of administrative continuity.

SPACE

The provision of space suggests the maintenance and commitment of an institutional or agency staff, and a relationship to other functions within the setting. It also extends the concept of sanction and implies that there has been some consideration given to logistical thinking regarding the total life of patients and clients in the setting.

EQUIPMENT

The acquisition of supplies and a variety of equipment for use in the program indicates budget commitments and the interaction of various staff personnel. Not only does it further extend the concept of sanction, but it offers tangible evidence of the institution's intent to potential program participants.

COORDINATION

This factor indicates the recognition of the relationship of recreation sponsorship to other activities that take place in the institution or agency, such as nursing care, dietetics, X-ray, physical therapy, social case work, vocational activity, counseling, and many others. It suggests an awareness of the demands made upon patient or client time and the necessity for positive personnel interaction. This factor also implies the involvement of groups from outside the institutional or agency complement, whose purpose may be to entertain, to educate, or to assist in some way. These groups are given the ability to conduct their involvement so that they move into and out of the structure in a precise manner.

Programming Methods

When one starts to develop a program, a number of models may be used. Some people use a "customary model" for planning purposes, feeling that what has been done by their predecessors has been accepted and is successful. When using this approach, they perpetuate and continue past activity elements, using these as the substance for their program. In some instances this approach may prove quite successful; however, program has a way of reflecting "administrative style" of the program director, and often when personnel changes do occur, this method proves faulty. This may be particularly apparent when the original program has been designed by an administrator who is an authoritarian personality and subsequently is directed by an administrator who is rather free and easy.

Some people use a "contemporary model" in program planning—observing what colleagues in similar settings do. They note the acceptance and success of elements in other settings, and then transplant those elements to their setting. They are alert to the content of professional journals and "graft" elements gleaned from these readings into their own program. Usually some modifications of elements observed in other settings or read about in journals must be undertaken before these elements function adequately in a different setting. At times this approach does not prove as successful as the original, because required modifications are often drastic, and program results become modified as well.

Certain egalitarian administrators prefer the "democratic model" in program planning, which requires surveying patient or client interest, using evaluative procedures after a new activity, interviewing new participants as to their likes and dislikes, and generally responding directly to participant requests and preferences. Program design becomes limited to "in-house" occupant awareness. Although as in the other schemes there is some merit to this approach, it is based on the assumption that potential participants are in a stable life situation, are knowledgeable regarding scope and range of possible recreation choices, and have access to logistical information regarding the setting and its variety of interacting services—often a faulty assumption.

Finally there is the "authoritarian model," which apparently draws its impetus from the "medical model." In this model, staff decisions are based upon staff interest and staff need with respect to professional goals and clinical considerations. This approach is often successful under certain circumscribed conditions, but is not generally applicable in all settings.

Perhaps no one method of program development is adequate in itself, and a combination or fusion of all models may be more productive. There are some customary aspects of program which have always proved successful in a given setting, and will remain successful because the setting is the crucial variable. Other customary elements cannot be perpetuated because of personnel changes, changes in popular taste, and clinical considerations. Gleaning the professional journals for ideas can be fruitful, as is an occasional observation of a similar setting. Through these means an administrator may find an alternative he has not thought about, and with judicious modification an idea may lend itself to his setting. Determining preferences of potential participants enables staff to remain aware of changes in taste, and sometimes may be used as a motivational factor. This also offers staff a clue to directions in which a program might be designed. However, this approach must also be viewed as a technique rather than the total method of program development, because in the final stage, the program director makes authoritative decisions—decisions based upon professional goals and clinical considerations rather than staff interest or personal desires.

The new program director can use a combination of all of these developmental models by examining existing program elements and modifying these in light of certain contemporary practices and potential participant preferences with respect to specific influential factors germane to the setting. These influential factors relate to the range of parameters that would be taken into consideration in planning program; namely, the nature of participants, administrative considerations, and of course treatment and care objectives.

The Nature Of Participants

INDIVIDUAL NEEDS

Although the raison d'etre for activity programming in therapeutic recreation service is considered to be based on a goal orientation with respect to a special setting rather than recreative experience per se, the recreation specialist recognizes that the patient or client does not check his needs at the door along with his personal possessions. It is also recognized that although therapeutic recreation service is primarily offered to persons who are ill, impaired, or disabled, this status is not a total human condition. Certain aspects of the total person are not affected by pathology, and individuals have need to be stimulated and exercised or they will suffer from secondary disability.

> This task of working out the best possible bargain between himself as a biological unit and himself as a social unit is not something that is accomplished at two or three or five and then forgotten. Nor is it sporadically accomplished at adolescence or in the late teens, never again presenting itself as a task or problem to be solved till mid-life or thereafter. The task of maintaining ... health (in its broadest terms) is *always* with us, and failure at any stage can make for unhappiness, inefficiency, and even ill health in the normal individual at the moment or can lay the foundation for future disabilities *based* upon these unfortunate responses of the moment.[2]

Many needs can be met through the recreation program, which can help to maintain those aspects of a total person that are still healthy. In effect, the recreation program may act as sustenance in a person's life, much in the manner of food and shelter. Needs are of different types—there may be need to be creative, or need to be of service. Some needs are expressed with the comment, "I've never been so unproductive for so long—I've got to do something!" Some needs may be unexpressed and often can be inferred from behavior. Needs act as a stimulus that motivates participation; therefore, it becomes imperative for the recreation specialist to determine whether or not there are "sustenance needs" of a special kind that can be met through recreation activity, and to determine whether or not these needs can be met through the current program content. Some needs are quite obvious and specific—if a person is hospitalized because of a broken left arm, he can still use his right arm and has physical need to use the rest of his body. If a person is institutionalized because of an intestinal infection, he can still think, talk, and probably has the use of both hands, although he might be bedbound for a time. If a person is institutionalized because he suffers from an anxiety reaction, he is physically able to engage in a broad range of activities; if a person is in a correctional institution, he usually faces no limitation other than a social one. If a person is homebound, he still has need for variable and interesting stimuli and socialization.

Thus program can take into account general needs of a health nature—that which will retain and strengthen healthy aspects of personality in any patient or client. The specialist must consider such areas as the needs for physical movement and exercise, intellectual stimulation, and emotional satisfaction. Although this is particularly true of people who are institutionalized, it may also be true of persons who live in the community. Often persons with disability who live in the community have limited opportunities for recreation because of a variety of barriers. Recreative activity can help to meet a range of personal needs.

[2] George E. Gardner, "Mental Health Problems of Normal Individuals," *Texas Trends,* IV, No. 4 (1947), 3.

at a certain age, the need for satisfactions in the other domains is not dormant, though it may be less demanding. Although the younger child requires considerable sensory-motor activity, he still has cognitive needs, and though the older child (perhaps 7 to 10 years of age) may have strong cognitive needs, he still requires sensory-motor gratification. Similarly, the older adult may have strong needs for affective gratification but still require some cognitive stimulation and sensory-motor activity.[4]

GENDER

There is much in the popular literature to suggest that whether one is male or female, activity participation with respect to gender is culturally determined rather than biologically ordained, and gender is not really an important consideration in recreation. However, if one programs in a culture that distinguishes some activities as "male activities" and other as "female activities," one must take gender into account. An example of cultural determination is contained in the following:

> In a home for elderly persons it was noted that during a game of poker in which both men and women were playing, Mrs. Rastt did not bet on the last card. When a new recreation specialist asked her why she didn't bet, since she could have changed the status of the game, Mrs. Rastt with some surprise replied, "Why only men can bet on the last card!"

There are indeed some distinct physical and emotional factors that differ with respect to gender in such areas as strength, temperament, and dexterity, to name a few. These differences are biological, and are not culturally determined. For example, females become better coordinated earlier in their lives than do males. This does not mean that certain activities should be viewed for men or women only—but rather suggests differences in participation style, and program should be structured accordingly. There are obvious physical differences with respect to singing in a choir, or engaging in a variety of gymnastic and tumbling activities, but there are also subtle manual differences with respect to certain crafts and other manipulative activities. In addition, many women experience mood changes during the menstrual cycle which effect their activity participation. Thus the factor of gender does need to be considered in program development.

ETHOS

This factor may not only be important with respect to what men or women may or may not do, but is quite influential in the total choice of activity. Mores, prejudices, customs, folkways, goodwill—all influence participa-

[4] See Alfred L. Baldwin, *Theories of Child Development* (New York: John Wiley and Sons, 1967); and James E. Birren, *Handbook of Aging and the Individual* (Chicago: University of Chicago Press, 1959).

Social and Behavioral Factors in Program Development

Each activity has peculiar *qualities* which appeal to certain individuals and which are important factors in the program. But its *values* need not be peculiar to the activity; many of the same values can result from activities which, on the surface, seem to be very different. This is due in part to the ability of individuals and groups to adapt activities to their needs. Prominent among these values are the potentialities for aiding physical growth and neuromuscular control and for providing intellectual stimulation and development. The release of emotions is also made possible, for the activities provide forms through which feeling may be acceptably expressed. And the activities further contribute patterns and disciplines which influence and limit behavior and provide security for members by indicating the kind of behavior expected.[3]

The following material offers the specialist engaged in program planning a deeper understanding of individual human differences and their relationship to recreation participation. Areas under consideration are chronological age, gender, ethos, socioeconomic status, educational status, life styles, and interests and skills.

CHRONOLOGICAL AGE

Activity interests change with age. The younger a participant is, the shorter his interest span and the less defined his leisure pattern and style. Growth and development proceeds in a hierarchical order with respect to the three behavioral domains.† First, there is growth and development in the sensory-motor domain, and after this domain reaches a plateau, growth and development begins in the cognitive domain. Subsequently, when the cognitive domain has reached a plateau, growth and development begins in the affective domain and the process is repeated until maturity. Thus at any given age, there is an imbalance in the three behavioral domains until maturity, but the concept of maturity is relative and an abstract notion, particularly in the cognitive and affective domains. In old age, decline is not uniform and the process is similar to the growth pattern in early life; that is, imbalance in the three domains. An older person may experience some physical decline but no decline in the cognitive or affective domain. Subsequently there may be decline in the cognitive domain, such as memory loss, but a retarding of sensory-motor decline at this time. It is perhaps more logical to consider chronicity with respect to development or decline in the behavioral domains rather than with respect to years of life. In any event, within certain age ranges there is a need and demand for a predominance of sensory-motor activity; within other age ranges there is a primary need and demand for cognitive stimulation; and within still other age ranges there is a readiness for deeper affective gratifications. Although one domain predominates

---

[3] Gertrude Wilson and Gladys Ryland, *Social Group Work Practice* (Cambridge, Mass.: Houghton Mifflin Co., 1949), p. 153.
† For detailed discussion of the behavioral domains, see Chapter ii.

tion. Although an activity in reality is neutral, it wears (in Margaret Mead's terms) certain "cultural clothes." A recreation specialist may view activity in the context of a "stripped universal," but to participants activities do indeed suggest "the people across the river," "our crowd," "not for us," and other familiar ethnic expressions. The more ethnocentricity present in a given setting, the more a program becomes dominated by this factor, and recreation specialists might take this into account to insure participation. Ethos influences activity in specific ways. For example, it may function to exclude certain activities such as gambling or costume parties in a certain setting, or it may require that nourishment be present at each activity for the activity to be considered successful by participants. Ethos may foster the purchase of certain types of equipment such as a "schafkopf" card deck (a special German card game) or recordings of "bouzouki" music (a Greek folk instrument). Ethos may mitigate against certain types of tours that require eating different foods, or negate participation in service activities that carry social class connotations. Ethos may encourage participation in certain holiday celebrations and discourage participation in others. Ethos can be a powerful determinant in program content, depending upon the setting and its population.

SOCIOECONOMIC STATUS

A knowledge of the socioeconomic status (SES) of the patient or client population often enables the recreation specialist to anticipate participation patterns and styles. There is considerable information in the literature that indicates that there are differences in activity preferences and involvement of people in different economic strata of society. Likes in theater, television, motion pictures, magazines, and other media are well-documented. There is some evidence regarding differences in types of sport and game involvement and a number of other popular recreative activities. Data is available concerning the relationship between various SES groups and attendance at or viewing of specific professional sports on television. All of these subtle differences can be noted and used in the process of program development. A predominance of one stratum in a setting will necessitate program plans that include activities usual within that stratum, while a setting that serves people from a number of socioeconomic strata should offer a broader range of activity choices. A recreation specialist must caution against planning a program based upon the SES of personnel rather than patient or client SES. This can not only limit patient or client participation but can also encourage unrealistic expectations on the part of participants, and may have the effect of depressing them, and in some instances, provoking anxiety.

EDUCATIONAL STATUS

Closely allied to SES is educational status. There is considerable evidence to indicate that persons with more formal education have more varied leisure interests and a greater knowledge of activity choice than do persons with less formal education. Often those with more formal education not only have accumulated more knowledge about what activities are available in society at large, but they often know in which activities they find greater satisfaction. Persons with little formal education have limited knowledge of the broad range of recreations and consequently have a limited leisure pattern. This is not to say that persons with less formal education may not be stimulated to explore a new activity, but it suggests that the specialist cannot assume they have had considerable experience in recreation. Thus if the patient or client population is educationally homogeneous, program planning on this dimension may prove relatively simple (given that staff is not dealing with a more educated group than itself). On the other hand, most settings cater to persons who are educationally heterogeneous and thus it becomes necessary to identify levels of education in the patient or client population and plan accordingly. It is also important that planning not focus on the "average" level of education in a setting, but try to offer elements that span the educational range present in the patient or client population.

LIFE STYLES

In recent years, social and behavioral scientists working for commercial segments of the leisure service industry have been conducting research concerning participants and their lives—research that goes beyond the usual demographic classifications. Demographic classifications are some of the variables that have been discussed thus far, and include age, gender, ethos, SES, and education. These variables may be viewed as being along a horizontal axis, segmenting a population into various groups that have certain common traits. These traits or characteristics can tell the recreation specialist a number of things that are useful in program planning. However, they do not offer any clues regarding the intensity of participation or the likelihood of continued participation and other similar factors. In other words, demographic information does not indicate depth, or a vertical axis regarding participation or "consumption." Thus, researchers in the commercial sector of the leisure service industry have begun to identify aspects of this vertical axis. These aspects are referred to in the literature as psychographics, or life style phenomena. For example. with respect to tourism, and particularly tourists who fly, data from depth interviews indicate that these people may be divided into three major groups—those who fly a great deal, heavy fliers; those who fly a little, light fliers; and those who usually don't fly. The heavy fliers are identified as having an "allocentric life style," and the nonflyers as having a "psychocentric life style." The following chart indicates life style differences in the allocentric and psychocentric style:

Social and Behavioral Factors in Program Development

ALLOCENTRIC	PSYCHOCENTRIC[5]
travel-oriented	sense of powerlessness
anxiety-free	anxious/nervousness
interested/involved	nonactive
adventurous	nonadventurous
self-confident	lacking confidence
curious	restrictive
risk-taker	non-risk-taker
uses income	withholds income
tries new things	uses traditional things
explores	territory-bound

Another example is concerned with examining life style with regard to reading habits. In a series of large-scale studies, Wells has identified five life styles:[6]

Self-indulgent pleasure-seeker has a routine, uninteresting job, satisfaction comes from real or imagined action and adventure out of doors; prefers outdoor sports and powerful cars; is an impulse buyer and heavy credit user; always short of cash; doesn't make long-range plans; doesn't read much, but is heavy viewer of sports, action, and adventure programs on television.

Active achiever in pursuit of upward mobility, is interested in his employment; liberal and contemporary and has opinions on many subjects; sure of self and skills; seeks new experiences of many kinds; is interested in such activities as sailing, skiing, foreign travel; reads to keep abreast of current events and latest trends in popular culture; watches sports programs, talk shows, and news analysis on television.

Executive (the active achiever who has "arrived"); purchases club memberships, vacations, second homes; less geographically mobile and involved with family activity; reads business magazines and news magazines; views news and news analysis, travel specials, and nature specials on television.

Blue collar strong beliefs in conventional values; primacy of patriotism, morality, and hard work; activities include hunting, fishing, and family camping; on television watches such things as bowling and pro football.

---

[5] W. A. Garrett, "Life Style and Psychographic Analysis of the Air Traveler," Proceedings of the Third International Travel Research Conference, Quebec City, 1972.

[6] W. D. Wells, *Life Styles in Selecting Media for Travel Advertizing,* paper presented at the 1972 International Travel Research Conference, Quebec City, Canada, August 15. See also R. J. Havinghurst and K. Feigenbaum, "Leisure and Life Style," *American Journal of Sociology* (January 1959), 64, pp. 396-404.

Traditional homebody old-fashioned, tries to wring the greatest value from every dollar; avoids anything that is fancy, frivolous, risky, or extravagant; watches situation comedy on television, and uses early evening news as major source of information about national and world events.

Life-style analysis research attempts to get attitudes, values, interests, opinions, personality traits, perceptions, and activity preferences of participants. Although demographic analysis is quantitative, life-style analysis is qualitative. Life-style analysis is not based on theories, but makes use of extensive depth interviews and psychological testing with large population samples. Standard life-style testing materials are beginning to be made available for general use. Thus, as more life style analytic information becomes available, it will assist recreation personnel in general to more adequately plan program content. The therapeutic recreation specialist can use the life-style analysis technique to qualitatively understand the patient or client population for which he is providing program services.

INTEREST AND SKILL

A program failing to offer elements that include patient or client interests is a program that will experience low levels of participation. It is important to determine which activity elements interest clients and which do not. Similarly, it is necessary to determine which elements generate high levels of interest and which are engaged in because there is nothing better to do with one's time. Activities calling for high levels of skill can only be incorporated if these levels of skill are present in the patient or client group. For example, the setting may include opulent resources for dramatic presentations, but if enough interest is not present in the patient or client group, the setting can just as well not have these resources. A specialist may determine that "live music" at various functions would increase effectiveness, but unless there are patients or clients who have enough musical skill to play for an audience, such a plan is not feasible. It is necessary to determine how much knowledge patients and clients have about recreation activities and at what level is their capacity to participate. Are they beginners, or do they know more about an activity than any member of the staff? It is not necessary to base all program elements upon patient or client interest, because new and different elements often act as a stimulus, and many people are anxious to learn new things. However, some elements in a program must be based on client interest, not only to insure participation, but because they offer a frame of reference that provides for familiarity and stability—something necessary to persons in a strange setting.

In questioning adult participants in a long-term care institution about types of activities which hold interest for them, the following facts were indicated:

Social and Behavioral Factors in Program Development

Most people stated they would prefer activities that offered opportunities to get out rather than stay in. This would indicate that a general interest could be maintained in the world at large if a portion of a recreation program offered in a congregate living situation included use of community resources and facilities rather than a complete program within the institutional setting. Such activities as a weekly leisurely drive through the community with a stop at a famous landmark, or a more elaborate trip to a special activity such as a concert, a tea, or an exhibit could be undertaken. However, this experience is not valuable when it is done with fifty people at a time. Interest is in such activity with five or six persons—the usual number of people that engage in this type of social activity as a group. In addition, less ambulant persons indicate that they have more need to have at least one opportunity every few months to get out.

Second to getting out, participants reported that they would like something in their monthly routine that is different and special rather than the same thing all the time. It is interesting to note that commercial television has found it necessary to have "specials" to maintain audience interest. Everyone likes a little spice in his life, and persons in institutions who are subjected to the same routine day after day need change more intensely. When questioned about what might be considered special, participants indicated that this might be a special meal, or meeting someone with whom they wouldn't ordinarily come into contact, or attending a social function that is varied and different from others they attend.

The third reported area was to have opportunities to follow an individual bent rather than having to be consistently one of the crowd. Some participants indicated that this could mean having the freedom to choose pictures or a color scheme every few months in order to change the look of their rooms. Others indicated it might mean having a bath or shower in the evenings as they had been doing before institutionalization, even though this is contrary to institutional routine. Most participants, though, indicated that it means engaging in a hobby that is often not offered in the organized recreation program. Some indicated that they would appreciate the opportunity to have a glass of port or a highball in the evening before retiring.

A fourth area involved the request of keeping involved rather than losing touch. Participants requested opportunities to be informed about what is going on outside the institution. Some indicated the desire to have political candidates invited to come and speak about their policies, or other newsworthy personages and groups to come to tell their side of the story. Some suggested the scheduling of a special session after viewing certain televised events in order to discuss the ramifications of the events. Others indicated that modified newpapers with large print should be available for those who have difficulty with vision, and that volunteers should be available regularly to read to those who cannot see.

A fifth area concerned contributing rather than being dependent. A variety of examples were offered by participants, such as being the eyes of another who cannot see, establishing a committee to assist in the selection of motion pictures, arranging flowers for religious services, and many others. Some participants indicated that they needed to be visibly productive and suggested such interests as the manufacture of tray favors and table centerpieces to be used throughout the institution. It was strongly agreed that no one likes to be involved in making useless items, and all manufacture should have immediate utility if it is to be satisfying.

Other responses indicated that some participants would like to continue to learn—some indicated a desire to learn another language, more about history, and the meaning of current political events. It was suggested that these learning experiences did not have to be in large weekly formal classes, but rather in small informal sessions with a few people and a person from outside the institution who has knowledge and a desire to share this knowledge with others.

Some indicated that they wished there were some excitement and adventure in their lives because they were bored, while others craved the familiar and the comfortable rather than the strange and new. Some wanted opportunity to engage in activities that are natural and creative for adults in today's world rather than the number of artificial and childlike activities often offered to them. Finally, some participants requested that the recreation program help to keep them in touch with reality rather than encouraging daydreaming and fantasy.

It becomes apparent from these responses in an institutional setting that interest is less tied to specific activities than to the motives of participants and the values they ascribe to activities. It behooves the recreation specialist to understand this concept when examining patient or client interests and skills in a specific setting.

Administrative Considerations

There are many texts concerned with the administration of service, but few examine the influence of administrative variables with respect to program planning in recreation and ultimately the influence of these variables upon participation. In the following, specific administrative aspects will be examined in this light; namely, factors in the setting such as location, climate, space, time, census, manpower, and finance.

THE INSTITUTION

In 1854, Thomas Kirkbride, superintendent of the Pennsylvania Hospital in Philadelphia, published his ideas concerning the organization of hospitals and related institutions. Institutions constructed and organized in relation to his concepts were known thereafter as Kirkbride hospitals, and were based upon the principle that a hospital should not be larger than the capacity of the administrator to remember the first name of all staff and patients! Kirkbride

Social and Behavioral Factors in Program Development 119

believed in "moral treatment" and encouraged trips, lectures, outdoor activities, arts and crafts, and a host of other services for patients. He felt that no hospital should be constructed without some area devoted to gardens and pleasure-grounds for patients.[7]

Kirkbride's concepts ran the gamut of administrative concerns—from the plumbing facilities to the organization of the board of trustees. His thoughts had much to do with the structure and operations of institutions, particularly long-term care institutions in North America for over a hundred years. It would be unfair, however, to lay all of the problems of these institutions at Kirkbride's feet, because many institutional administrators and the groups to which they were responsible did not entirely follow his concepts. Many other intervening factors also influenced the nature of hospitals and related institutions. A little more than a hundred years later, Goffman, in studying hospitals, noted their similarity to other kinds of social institutions and coined the phrase "total institutions." Some of the characteristics of living in a total institution follow:

- There are barriers to social interaction outside the institution;
- There is a tendency to sleep, play, and work in the same place with the same set of participants, under the same authority, with a rational plan;
- All aspects of life are conducted in the same place, under the same single authority, in the company of a large group, all the members of which are treated alike;
- All activity is tightly scheduled, with one activity leading at a pre-arranged time to the next;
- All activity is imposed from above through a system of explicit rulings;
- Activity forms a single overall rational plan to fulfill official aims of the institution;
- The handling of many human needs is accomplished by bureaucratic organization of whole blocks of people;
- Because blocks of people move in time, only a relatively small number of supervisory personnel is needed;
- One person's infraction of the rules is likely to stand out in relief against the visible, constantly examined compliance of others;
- Patients and clients have restricted contact with staff who are integrated into the outside world.

This is indeed a bleak picture and has many implications for recreation personnel. Goffman further indicates:

> In the ordinary arrangements of living in our society, the authority of the work-place stops with the worker's receipt of a money payment; the spending of this in a domestic and recreational setting is at the discretion of the worker and is the mechanism through which the authority of the work-place is kept within strict bounds. However, to say that inmates in total institutions have their full day scheduled for them is to say that some

---

[7]Thomas Kirkbride, *On the Construction, Organization, and General Arrangements of Hospitals,* 1st ed. 1854, 2nd ed. 1880. For a review and reprinting of some of the chapters from Kirkbride's book see Charles E. Goshen, *Documentary History of Psychiatry* (New York: Philosophical Library, 1967), pp. 505-26.

version of all basic needs will have to be planned for too. In other words, total institutions take over "responsibility" for the inmate, and must guarantee to have everything that is defined as essential "layed on." It follows then, that, whatever incentive is given for work, this will not have the structural significance it has on the outside. Different attitudes and incentives regarding the central feature of our life will have to prevail. Here, then, is one basic adjustment required of those who work in total institutions, and those who must induce these people to work. In some cases, no work or very little is required, and inmates, untrained often in leisurely ways of life, suffer extremes of boredom.[8]

Goffman paints an even bleaker picture indicating that patients and clients go through a "rite of passage" which he calls the "stripping process"—a process which mortifies the patient or client and takes away his individuality and ego supports by divesting him of his personal property, including his clothes. Much of Goffman's work concerns long-term care institutions. In a series of studies concerning short-term institutions, Dichter showed many of the same findings. His study reports how hospitalization militates against a patient's feelings of security and how the hospital engenders feelings of helplessness and insecurity. Of particular importance to personnel concerned wth recreation service is the following:

> the hospital experience for the adult was not only threatening, but boring and frustrating as well..... The hospital must recognize the emotional value not only of attitudes but of activities. . . . It was found in the study that a large portion of the patients and former patients interviewed had their sense of insecurity, fear, and helplessness heightened by a lack of knowledge at every level. They did not know what to expect of themselves, of the treatment, of the staff, and so on..... Inactivity and loneliness, added to the patient's enforced dependency, also enhanced these feelings of postoperative depression..... The emotional strain of an "inactive" convalescence can be quite heavy, even when the convalescence is neither painful, serious, nor physically difficult..... A lack of information and enforced inactivity can threaten the security of a person hospitalized merely for observation..... The patient as he convalesces becomes increasingly a social being..... They constantly remembered the depressing effects of boredom, frustration, and lack of activity. While some hospitals were neutral in their attitude toward socialization among patients, and neither encouraged nor prevented it, others were violently opposed. The head nurse on the private floor of a medium-sized hospital said: "We discourage any social activity of our private patients. We discourage their coming to the lounge to sit. After all they are private patients. They might not want to talk to everyone..... It is not necessary for them to mingle with other people. Most of them need rest. Anyhow we have a high turnover among patients. They go home as soon as they

---

[8] Irving Goffman, "On the Characteristics of Total Institutions," *Asylums* (Garden City, N.Y.: Doubleday and Co., 1961); see also Samuel E. Wallace, *Total Institutions* (Washington, D.C.: Transactions, Inc., 1971).

possibly can." The study revealed though, that there is no distinction by class in the basic emotional needs of the patient..... the need for assurance, the need for sharing and return to maturity were common regardless of age, education, or class. . . . The patient, as he progresses in his convalescence, wishes for security. He hungers for anything that would make him feel secure. He wishes for something to do. But not simply, however, for some sterile time-consuming activity. He would prefer to feel that what he does has some value, either privately or socially.[9]

It must be recognized then, that in program planning, an institution is an entity that is primarily directed toward goals other than recreative experience. Its systems and procedures are calculated to enhance goals other than recreation. It is obvious from the work of Goffman, Dichter, and others that patients and clients must submerge their individuality at the expense of these systems. It is also somewhat obvious that the recreation program is perhaps the only "outpost" in an institution in which a patient or client can express his individuality. However, in order to offer this type of sanctuary it becomes necessary to plan a program that complements the various institutional systems and procedures. To these ends, certain aspects of the setting must be considered.

LOCATION

An institution in the heart of an urban area has access to a variety of rich resources which can augment program content. The recreation specialist can draw upon nearby community recreation facilities, commercial recreation facilities, sources for equipment, sources for entertainment, volunteers, and many other things. However, there are some problems attendant with being located in a densely populated urban area. In addition to the usual stresses and strains of urbanization, such issues as problems with public transport to and from the institution and daily visits of friends and relatives to the institution are but two aspects that will influence program. In contrast, when an institution is located away from an urban center it usually has its own means of transporting patients or clients to and from the setting. Also, friends and relatives are less likely to visit frequently and are less of a program concern. On the other hand, there are far fewer public and commercial recreation resources which the recreation specialist can draw upon in a suburban or rural area, and the securing of supplies, equipment, and volunteers is often problematic. Thus, where a setting is geographically located affects the recreation program.

CLIMATE

If a setting is primarily concerned with service to patients or clients who are physically disabled, climate becomes an important programming factor. A long season of warm weather makes outside activity feasible. On the other hand,

[9] Ernest Dichter, "The Hospital-Patient Relationship," a report originally published in the *Modern Hospital,* (September, October, November, December 1954 and January, February 1955).

if the climate is very warm or hot, this limits participation in certain types of activities, and limits certain patients who might be photosensitive because of medication or age. Institutions that are in colder climates and that have relatively long winters, of necessity need to consider intense indoor program plans for physically ill or disabled persons. In the event an institution is in a "long winter" climate and its patients or clients are not institutionalized for physical illness, a program plan would have to consider the use of winter activities outside. Swimming, which has recreative value and is often used for physical therapy as well as for its psychological implications, becomes problematic with respect to climate depending upon the availability of resources. Similarly, when climate is examined with regard to location, the question of the availability of resources becomes a major factor in planning.

SPACE

Most institutions do not have adequate recreation or social spaces. This is to be expected, because this is not the primary concern of the institution. Thus, in program planning, a recreation specialist must consider which indoor and outdoor space can be utilized for recreative purposes, regardless of any official designations for these areas. Can a dead-end hallway do double duty on some days as a bowling alley? Can a parking lot serve as a site for a carnival? Can the physical therapy clinic serve as a classroom in the evenings? Can the staff dining room accommodate a birthday party between lunch and supper? Can the social work conference room be turned into a language laboratory once a week? Can the fifth-floor dayroom be used for an indoor cookout? Can the nursing staff classroom double as a music room on weekends? These are the types of questions a recreation specialist would consider concerning space usage as he engages in program planning within an institution. However, some similar issues are of concern to the specialist in a nonresidential community setting as well. In both the residential and community settings, the specialist is concerned with the availability of space that can serve two or more simultaneous activities. There is also the question of the type of activity for the space—not just the size of the space, but how accessible it is for the numbers involved or the degree of participant disability. Another issue is the proximity of toilets, drinking water, a telephone for emergencies, and similar safety concerns. If an activity is noisy, will it interfere with other activities in adjacent spaces? It can be seen that space becomes a vital issue in program planning.

TIME

The public at large in all cultures develops its own rhythm for leisure involvement, and the leisure service industry responds to this rhythm. Theater and professional sports are offered to the public when they have unobligated time—usually in the evenings, on weekends, or on holidays. People usually have special meals in restaurants in the late afternoon or evening. Parties and dances are usually held in the late afternoon or evening. Gambling casinos open for business in the evening. Families entertain in their homes in the evenings and on weekends. Bridge games are played in the late afternoon or evening. Most people engage in hobby activity in the evening. Within Western civilization this is generally the pattern, with some slight variations. For example, during the summer, Norwegians are at work early in the morning, have a quick, light lunch, and an early dinner. They then engage in recreation from about 4:30 P.M. until late in the evening. This is done to make maximum use of the daylight hours in summer. In contrast, people in Greece and Spain work from about 8:00 A.M. until noon, and then take four or five hours to rest, swim, or socialize until 5:00 or 6:00 P.M. Then they return to work until 9:00 or 10:00 P.M. This pattern exists because of climate and tradition. In many Norwegian cities it is difficult to find a restaurant that will serve dinner *after* 6:00 P.M., while in Greece it is difficult to find a restaurant that will serve dinner *before* 10:00 P.M.

In an institutional complex, patients and clients are there 24 hours a day, 7 days a week. The rhythm of patients and clients is the rhythm of the institution. They awake when the morning shift comes on duty, be it 6:00 or 7:00 A.M., even if this is not their usual time of arising. There is much in the literature concerning the problem of the morning routine in institutions and the tyranny of the thermometer in the early morning. Meals are offered on a scheduled basis—not when a patient or client feels hungry. Usually the evening meal is lighter than the noon meal, and is served earlier than most people would want because of the way institutional staff time is structured. Clinic visits for physical therapy, X-ray, psychotherapy, and all the rest may be at the same time each day or they may be scheduled at various times throughout the day. In some cases, although a time is set in advance, all schedules are modified when there is a cancellation, regardless of what a patient or client is engaged in. As with all institutional structures, there is a considerable degree of "hurry up and wait." Some patients and clients have lengthy unobligated periods because they receive special treatments only once or twice a week, and in some cases even less frequently. In some settings, because the evening shift has less manpower than the day shift, not only are meals served earlier than usual, but often patients and clients who need special personal care are prepared for sleep before 6:00 P.M., and are unable to have access to public social places in that setting in the evenings.

Because of these patterns in time use, program planning becomes even more complex. Activity must be offered when patients or clients have unobligated time rather than at a time that is usual for certain leisure activities. However the time used must be realistic with regard to the activity. Because a patient or client has unobligated time from 8:30 to 11:30 A.M., it is not realistic to expect him to attend a dance at that time. Furthermore, because "time reality" within an institutional complex is different from that of the world outside—that is, the continuous nature of service, day in and day out throughout the year—it becomes important for recreation personnel to think with respect to recreation-time. Recreation time for most people is late afternoons and evenings, with Friday and Saturday evening being more special than the rest. Weekends are different from the rest of the week, and holidays are different from all other days. Birthdays and anniversaries are different from other days, as well. Recreation-time thinking is not based on the calendar months of the year, but on program periods that run from holiday to holiday, for example from Christmas to New Years' Day, or Valentine's Day to St. Patrick's Day, or Canada Day to Bastille Day. It then becomes the task of the recreation specialist to integrate the recreation-time with the institutional cycle, thus affording patients and clients a bridge with the world at large. Careful consideration must be given to time as an aspect of program planning.

CENSUS

An important administrative consideration in program planning is the number of patients or clients to be served in a given setting and the incidence of activity offerings to meet the needs of this number of potential participants. In theory, the recreation department is responsible for all persons in the setting, but in reality this is often not feasible. In short-term care settings, some persons are too ill to engage in recreative activity, while in long-term care settings some persons may not wish to be involved in an organized program. In settings serving persons who are extremely impaired, very minimal involvement in a recreation program is all that is possible. Certain activities lend themselves to use with different population groups, such as structures for individual involvement, while other activities can serve aggregates of patients or clients in small groups. Some activities are perfect for large group and mass involvement. In settings that tend to depersonalize "inmates," it is important to program individual and small-group experiences to enable patients and clients to maintain a sense of the personal. Some people however, find it satisfying to engage in large group and mass activities as well. Thus in planning, a balance must be struck in this aspect of programming, and as the census changes, so must the recreation program.

MANPOWER

In order to provide service, regardless of the number of potential participants or the types of elements to be incorporated into the program, it must be recognized that manpower would have to be available in residential care settings at times when participants have unobligated time each day of the week. Institutional service patterns cannot be based on the "leisure rhythms" present in society per se. Theoretically this means that recreation personnel would be on duty from perhaps eight in the morning until midnight, seven days a week. If one were to consider an average work day as seven or eight hours, this would mean that there would be two shifts of recreation personnel each day—8:00 A.M. until 4:00 P.M. and 4:00 P.M. until midnight. If the work week is to include 35 or 40 hours and to span five or six days per worker, this would mean a minimum of three personnel on a recreation staff per institution to have coverage in each time period. This does not allow for vacation time or holidays. Furthermore, as more individual, small-group, specialized service and simultaneous service is offered, the personnel picture changes and additional personnel are required. When planning for an institution with a large census, the personnel picture changes again in order to provide duplicate services to a large number of service recipients. As the number of personnel increases, some personnel are partially or completely withdrawn from direct service to patients or clients, and of necessity must be concerned with administrative and supervisory tasks. Depending upon the sophistication of the institution, direct service time also becomes limited by the necessity for interdepartmental conferences of various types, report writing, activity preparation, and evaluation. This latter aspect limits direct service even more, and alters the manpower picture. Finally, because of the extent of recreation activity itself, it is not possible for any one staff member to be knowledgeable in all activity areas nor to have leadership skill in all but a small number of activities. Thus, in program planning, the specialist must take into consideration not only how many personnel are available at specific times, but for which activities available personnel can take responsibility, how much time can be afforded each person for administrative tasks such as reports, preparation, conferences, and so forth, and how this time can be utilized most effectively to provide service to the largest numbers of patients or clients. The specialist must also concern himself with effective use of volunteer personnel in the same way he would consider employed personnel.

The manpower issue in community settings is somewhat similar, however —because service recipients reside in a place other than the agency, there is more likelihood that the agency will provide service within the "leisure rhythm" pattern of the community. There will be less pressure toward concern for universal coverage, or service to all in the community who need service. A community agency generally limits the population to which it provides service, while this is not possible in a residential setting.

FINANCE

In every endeavor, financial support is a crucial factor in the provision of service. In therapeutic recreation service, fiscal influences upon program become a leavening factor. Depending upon amounts available, the specialist must decide whether he can staff certain aspects of a program, if he can afford the cost of certain supplies or equipment as well as the rental of external service or space, and whether he can provide a quality program to the quantity of patients or clients who require service. Priorities must be determined, long-range plans for capital expenditure must be made, and relative values of different services must be determined.

Fortunately, therapeutic recreation service is in a position (because of the nature of recreation) to utilize alternative resources when there are budget constraints. Unlike many other service fields which cannot substitute activities, equipment, or personnel, therapeutic recreation service can often do this. For example, it is acknowledged that the largest portion of a program budget is personnel. Recreation service has traditionally augmented its program through the use of volunteers. Often, the word "volunteer" is inadequate to express the contribution of these "employees without fiscal compensation." Some volunteers are highly skilled and in reality could not be paid members of the staff because of budget limitations. Some persons in the field disagree with the concept of augmenting staff by using volunteers. They indicate that there should be sufficient funds in the budget to employ necessary staff personnel. This principle is stringently adhered to in some places, and in Goteberg, Sweden, for example, volunteers are not used in the recreation department of the large regional psychiatric hospital and in other similar settings. However, in many comparable institutions in Canada, the principle of volunteer use is well accepted, and a cadre of volunteers can be found in many institutions.

Other persons in the field do not make use of volunteers because they feel that the amount of supervision required causes a budgetary drain, and funds could be better spent by employing direct service personnel. Some feel that volunteers are not dependable and thus cause additional fiscal problems. However, many feel that volunteers enrich a program because of their expertise in various recreation activities, and their ability to strengthen normal social experiences of the patient or the client, and the fact that they represent reality and are not constrained by the institutional or agency system. These latter factors in most cases seem to outweigh the negative factors, and many recreation specialists indicate that no budget could include enough funds to purchase these attributes.

Another alternative resource that enlarges limited fiscal support for program is the fact that therapeutic recreation service personnel have community counterparts who are in a position to share a wealth of recreation resources without charge. These resources may be personnel, supplies, equipment, space, and program activities per se. Often there does not need to be capital expenditure for institutional recreation facilities because a community recreation department already has the facility and it can be used by the institutional or agency staff. Often program can be supplemented by libraries, museums, and other community agencies who are pleased to bring in their resources. . Finally, program budget can be augmented by business and industry. This may run the gamut from the provision of speakers and films for special events to a window display from a department store that forms the basis of party decorations during a holiday event.

Thus in program planning in therapeutic recreation service, although there may be fiscal constraints that tend to limit the scope of programs, the specialist is able to draw upon a host of community resources that can expand the funds he has available to him for his program.

This chapter has offered a variety of social and behavioral information to take into consideration when planning a therapeutic recreation service program. The following chapter explains in detail how a systems analysis technique may be applied in the field of therapeutic recreation service for purposes of program planning. The author is indebted to Dr. Carol Peterson for inclusion of this unpublished material on a systems approach to program planning.

9
Applications of Systems Analysis Procedures to Program Planning in Therapeutic Recreation Service

Carol A. Peterson*

Introduction

A system can be defined as an entity, conceptual or physical, which consists of interdependent parts. A system which displays activity is called a behavioral system and is subject to control by human beings.[1] Around us everywhere are entities and phenomena that can be interpreted as systems under this definition. The concept of purpose and interacting components seems to describe institutions, organizations, social groups as well as individual behavior patterns. Beyond these basic concepts are characteristics of systems such as flow, feedback, and constant change that enable more realistic comprehension of entities that are not static. Despite the idea of "institutionalization," most entities involving people and service are changing phenomena, and thus are more accurately described by models that incorporate change in their basic presentations. A static model of a basic system can be diagrammed as follows:

INPUTS → TRANSFORMATION PROCESS → OUTPUTS

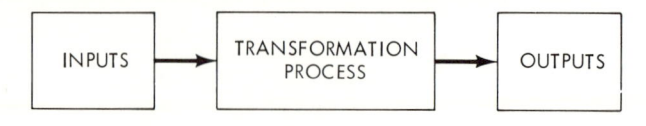

DIAGRAM I. FLOW PATTERN OF A SYSTEM[2]

---

* Reprinted with permission of the author.

[1] R. Ackoff, "Systems, Organizations, and Interdisciplinary Research," in *Systems: Research and Design,* ed. Donald Eckman (New York: John Wiley and Sons, Inc., 1961), pp. 27-28.

[2] Richard Hopeman, *Systems Analysis and Operations Management* (Columbus, Ohio: Charles E. Merrill Publishing Co., 1969), p. 16.

Application of Systems Analysis Procedures to Program Planning 129

This model implies that the inputs (some combination of clients, resources, personnel, materials, machines) pass through some transformation process (service perhaps) requiring the interaction of basic components, and the result is the output (changed behavior). However this basic flow model is static in that no feedback or adjustment mechanism is apparent.

A second model serves to illustrate a simple dynamic system with a feedback loop.

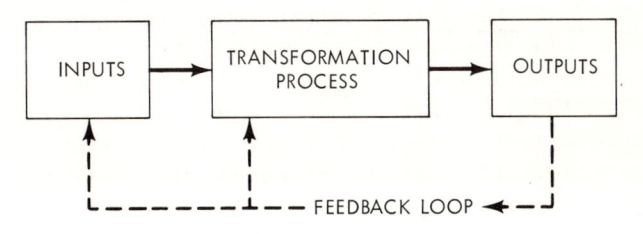

DIAGRAM II. FLOW PATTERN OF A SYSTEM WITH A FEEDBACK LOOP

The basic arrangement diagrammed here implies that the results of the system (the output) is used to change the nature of the input (and thus the nature of the total system) if performance does not measure up to expectations. In other words, if the outcome does not meet the objectives of the system, the system changes to adjust. Output can also be used to verify that the system is meeting its objectives. This concept of flow, feedback, and change is basic to the conceptualization of any entity as a system.

A system can also be depicted as having three basic aspects which are essential to the transformation process of the input-transformation-output scheme. These aspects can be identified as purpose, process, and content.

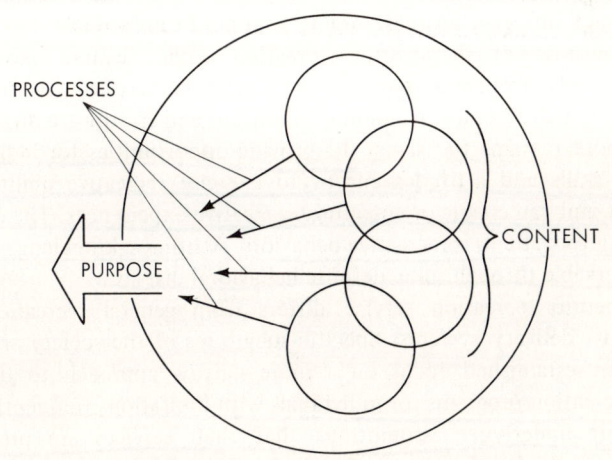

DIAGRAM III. ASPECTS OF A SYSTEM[3]

[3] Bela Banathy, *Instructional Systems* (Palo Alto, California: Fearon Publishers, 1968), p. 5.

Systems are made up of components or elements; the combination or sum of these may be called content. Each component is included in the system because it contributes in some way to the overall purpose of the system. To accomplish the purpose or purposes, different components engage in processes to bring about the intended transformation. This can be diagrammed on p. 129.

Therapeutic recreation service has been defined as "a specialized division of recreation service that is concerned with the provision of recreation programs for those people who have physical, mental, social, or chronological limitations." As such it most frequently takes administrative form and structure in organizations, agencies, or departments that provide programs to clients or service recipients. The conceptualization of these phenomena as a system requires the identification of the purpose of the system, the components, their processes, the nature of their interactions, the environment surrounding the system, the subsystems, and some of the basic characteristics of the behavior of the system.

Purpose of the System

Therapeutic recreation serves patients or clients who because of mental, physical, social, or chronological limitations are inhibited or prohibited from utilizing existing recreation resources. These individuals may reside in the community or in institutions. Their disabilities range in degree of severity and encompass numerous classifications within the broad categories mentioned above. Many have multiple problems such as the older resident of a nursing home who has both a physical disability as well as an isolating social situation, or the young child who is mentally retarded and lives in a family whose indifference contributes to the barriers already presented by his mental state. Determining a purpose for the therapeutic recreation service system must therefore be broad and inclusive, spanning a multitude of diverse programs, existing in many different settings, serving a variety of individuals.

The purpose of therapeutic recreation service cannot, however, be separated entirely from the purpose of recreation services for the normal individual, although several surrounding conditions and factors are different. The general purpose remains the same: To provide opportunities for individuals to gain leisure skills and attitudes and/or to exercise recreative abilities which already exist and can enable or encourage recreative experiences. The end result, product, or output, then, is recreative behaviors. Attitudes, knowledge, and skills must be observable through some definite behavioral display.

Therapeutic recreation service differs from general recreation service basically in its delivery systems. Specific subgroups of the society are selected and programs established focus on a more narrow approach to the overall purpose. Recreation programs for individuals with limitations frequently state or have as their underlying assumptions that their services are preventative, sustaining, or remedial in nature. These more specific functions imply that recreation services can be designed and implemented for a variety of purposes without losing sight of the long-range or ultimate goal, which is "enabling or encouraging recreative experience."

Application of Systems Analysis Procedures to Program Planning

Furthermore, many individuals with limitations require other service prior to, or in conjunction with therapeutic recreation service. Often the settings in which therapeutic recreation programs exist are multiservice settings, such as hospitals or comprehensive community mental health centers. The purpose of therapeutic recreation service in these settings then must be broad enough to encompass or contribute to the goals of a total service program.

An expanded statement of purpose can thus be stated as follows: *The purpose of a therapeutic recreation service system is to provide opportunities for individuals with limitations to gain leisure skills and attitudes, and/or to exercise recreative abilities within a framework of preventative, sustaining, or remedial services in order to enable or encourage recreative experience.*

It must be kept in mind that this is a general statement including all facets of the therapeutic recreation service system. A statement of purpose for a specific program in a given therapeutic recreation agency would, by necessity, be more definitive.

Nature of the System

The therapeutic recreation service system can be characterized in terms of inputs, the transformation process, and outputs. Inputs can be defined as "Whatever becomes subject to the system, or the material upon which the system operates."[4] In the case of the therapeutic recreation service system, the inputs would include the patients or clients and the resources available to the institution or agency; i.e., equipment, materials, facilities, knowledge and skills, financial assets, etc. The transformation process converts or acts on the input of the system. In therapeutic recreation, the different services the agency offers are the components or content of the transformation stage. Each component has a process (or processes) to accomplish its objective. It is the engagement of the service recipient in the processes of the different components that makes up the transformation function. The output is the resulting behavior of the client and can be stated in generalized terms for a comprehensive therapeutic recreation system. At this point "recreative behaviors" would most likely serve as the proper term. For a specific agency, a more definite description of the behavioral outcome would be required. This total process described above can be diagrammed as follows:

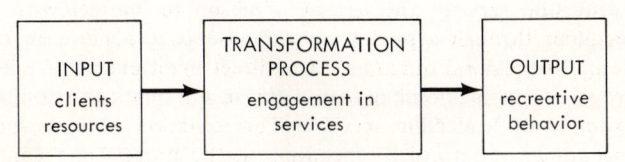

INPUT	TRANSFORMATION PROCESS	OUTPUT
clients resources	engagement in services	recreative behavior

DIAGRAM IV. BASIC FLOW PATTERN FOR THE THERAPEUTIC RECREATION SERVICE SYSTEM

[4] Ibid., p. 28.

In a conceptualization of a broad entity such as therapeutic recreation service, it is difficult to illustrate the nature of the feedback mechanism and system adjustment. The concept and process of feedback will be dealt with in detail in the following material in which a systems analysis program planning procedure is presented. Feedback, at that point, is central to the evaluation of the system's ability to meet its own specific objectives and purposes. For this conceptualization, it is important to note that the therapeutic recreation system is a dynamic and changing phenomenon. Over time, the nature of the output affects the environment of the system, and as a consequence, the nature of the inputs change (quantitatively at least) and result in the gradual sophistication, elaboration, and improvement of the transformation process.

Components and Processes

The specific services an institution or agency provides can be considered the components of the therapeutic recreation system. Although each may design its components somewhat differently, a taxonomy for service is offered to classify and present a comprehensive view of existing and possible components for a therapeutic recreation system. This classification attempts to be inclusive of all services described in the literature, yet remains flexible enough to accomodate new services which may be developed in the future.

Service provided to patients or clients may be classified as follows:

1. Administrative service: the provision of space, facilities, and/or equipment to be utilized by the service recipient. (Chess, checker sets, cards, or a television placed in the lounge area would be an example of an administrative service.) Function would be preventative, sustaining, or possibly remedial.
2. Supervisory service: the use of a person to act in a regulatory capacity in such matters as the concern for safety of the service recipients or maintenance of equipment. Interaction between the supervisor and the service recipient is minimal and is not designed in terms of clinical or therapeutic benefit. (An example of supervisory service would be the showing of a movie to service recipients with personnel present as overseers for safety or well-being). This service would probably be preventative or sustaining in function, but conceivably may be remedial.
3. Leadership service: the use of a person to interact with the service recipient through a predetermined process to achieve an expected or desired behavioral outcome. (The direct involvement of a leader and a group of nursing-home residents during a dramatics session would be an example of leadership service.) This function could be preventative, sustaining, or remedial depending on the process and content of the process design.
4. Educational service: the use of a person to expand knowledge, skill, or attitudes through the interaction with service recipients. (Leisure counseling with a soon-to-be discharged physical rehabilitation patient, or the teaching of a new recreative skill to a mentally retarded youth

Application of Systems Analysis Procedures to Program Planning

would be examples of this kind of service.) The function could be preventative, sustaining, or remedial.

This classification makes possible a minimum of twelve different therapeutic recreation services (a matrix of preventative, sustaining, remedial, administrative, supervisory, leadership, and educational services. The total program of the therapeutic recreation service system can thus be portrayed with the following model:

P1	P2	P3	P4	P∞
S1	S2	S3	S4	S∞
R1	R2	R3	R4	R∞

P preventative
S sustaining
R remedial
1 administrative
2 supervisory
3 leadership
4 educational

DIAGRAM V. MATRIX OF
THERAPEUTIC RECREATION SERVICES

It is unlikely that any given institution or agency would have all twelve prototype services. In most cases, however, they would provide more than one kind of service. Indeed it is quite possible for the program of a given organization to contain one type of service with several variations. This is possible since each service or component has an associated process. A given institution or agency determines the exact method or interaction procedure to be utilized in carrying out the specific service. For example, leadership-remedial service could have many variations as determined by the different interaction techniques and media available. In the design of new services using the proposed systems analysis technique, definitive descriptions of the actual interaction process for each service would be required in order to evaluate the effectiveness of the service. The flexibility in the selection of the interaction process or method for an individual service allows a wider choice of alternatives in the design of new programs, even if it is not helpful in classifying existing programs. For purposes of conceptualization of the total therapeutic recreation service system, it is sufficient to state that a comprehensive program is comprised of specific services and that these services can be represented by the matrix described above.

Subsystems and Integration of Components

In systems terminology, any arbitrarily selected set of interacting variables can be considered a system. This concept implies that the system under investigation is part of a larger system (the suprasystem) and that the system in question also contains subsystems.[5] Each component or service of the

---

[5] Donald P. Eckman, *Systems: Research and Design* (New York: John Wiley and Sons, Inc., 1961), p. ix.

therapeutic recreation system can therefore be considered a subsystem. As such, each subsystem contributes to the overall purpose of the total system in some distinct and yet integral way. The subsystem can be viewed as having its own lesser purpose and separate set of objectives and its own processes. Each subsystem can be separated and analyzed in detail, much the same way that the total system is discussed in this presentation. Subsystems do not exist in isolation. Banathy states, "The effectiveness of the system depends on how well the subsystems are integrated and how well they interfunction."[6] Therefore, it is important to include only those subsystems that contribute to the overall accomplishment of the system, yet fit or function within the context of the other subsystems.

When reviewing the total therapeutic recreation system each of the previously discussed services is included because of the potential each has to contribute to the ultimate purpose—that of enabling or encouraging recreative experience. The integration that exists is primarily a conceptual one, of contribution to a single goal.

In terms of a specific therapeutic recreation program in a given setting, the components or subsystems need to be integrated in a more distinct manner. Interaction and integration of the components is dependent upon a clearly stated purpose, carefully designed objectives, and processes for each subsystem, effective staff functioning, and continual assessment of the performance of the system. Procedures must be established to facilitate functional information transfer between services to insure unified direction toward the system's goals. A simple diagram of interlocking circles within a larger circle can be utilized to illustrate the interrelationship between subsystems and their enclosure within the larger system.

The Suprasystem and the Environment

The therapeutic recreation service system exists within the boundaries of a larger system, that system being the institution or agency, organization, or department that sponsors it. An organization may have several functions outside of the direct service to patients or clients, thus a separation of systems must be identified. This larger system will be referred to as the therapeutic recreation *agency* system. It has as its suprasystem, the society. The therapeutic recreation *service* system is directly influenced by its agency, the agency system in turn is influenced by the suprasystem. Likewise, the therapeutic recreation service system and its agency system influence the society through its outputs. This concept can be summarized by stating that the therapeutic recreation service system exchanges information with its environment, thus making it an open and adaptive system.

[6] Banathy, *Instructional Systems*, p. 6.

Application of Systems Analysis Procedures to Program Planning

Three relationships between the system and the suprasystem are identified by Banathy in regard to the educational system. These three conditions are also appropriate for the therapeutic recreation service system. Briefly they are as follows: (1) The suprasystem provides the input for the system in issue. In the case of the therapeutic recreation service system, the clients and all resources are supplied by the suprasystem, the agency. Indirectly the purpose and the resources, as well as the clients, come from the agency's suprasystem, society. The agency system receives the outputs of the service system, consequently the service system must produce an output that is acceptable to the agency. The same is true in regard to the society's acceptance or rejection of the agency's outputs. (2) The suprasystem also imposes constraints on the system in terms of the resources allotted. Normally, the resources allowed are less than sufficient to optimize the desired operation of the system. Nevertheless, the system in issue is judged by how well it uses the resources available. (3) The agency system must be aware of and sensitive to changes in the society or suprasystem.[7] For example, in the last ten years, society has become increasingly concerned with its responsibility for its members with limitations. The agency system and consequently the service system has therefore had the opportunity to utilize this change and adjust many of its programs to accommodate the increased demands, plus the chance to expand the range and scope of its service. The relationship between the therapeutic recreation service system, the therapeutic recreation agency system, and the suprasystem (society), can be diagrammed as follows:

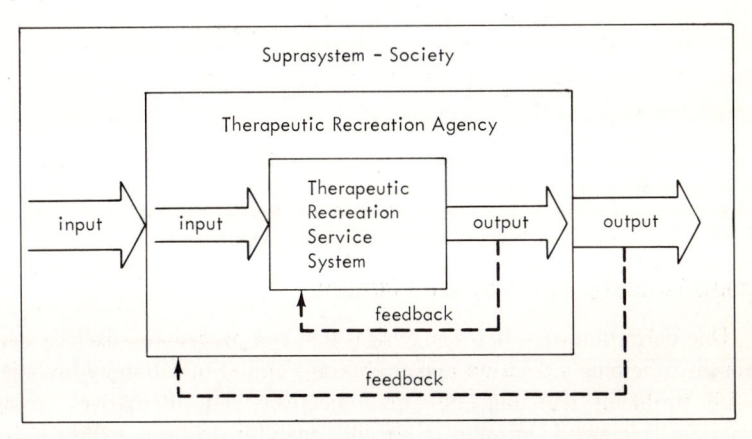

DIAGRAM VI. THERAPEUTIC RECREATION
SERVICE SYSTEM AND ITS SUPRASYSTEMS

The therapeutic recreation service system is also influenced by and in turn influences its peer service systems. Immediately surrounding the therapeutic recreation service system are the education, health, and community recreation

[7] Ibid., p. 10.

service systems. Constant flow of information and influence exist between these service systems. In some cases, the overlap is so great that it is impossible to determine the identification of a separate system.

Several other larger systems surround and influence the therapeutic recreation service system and its immediate peer service systems in both direct and indirect ways. These systems are government, business, and religion. The values of society indicated by the support these systems supply are vital to the maintenance of the therapeutic recreation system. A model of the therapeutic recreation service system and its environment is presented below.

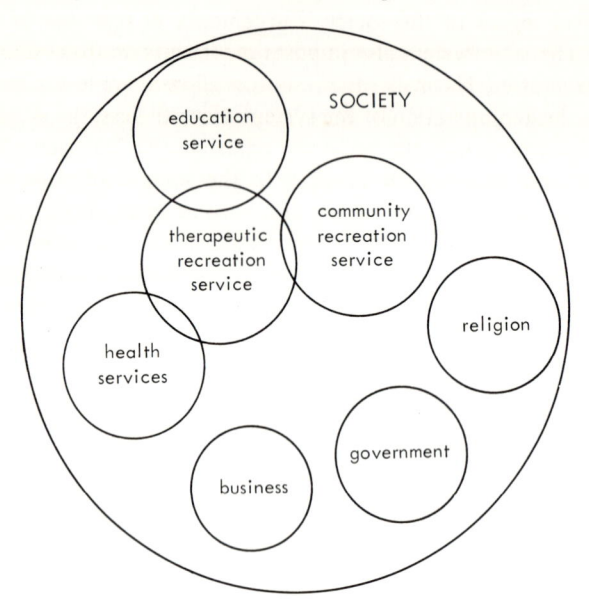

DIAGRAM VII. THERAPEUTIC RECREATION SERVICE SYSTEM AND ITS ENVIRONMENT

Systems Analysis and Program Planning

One definition of systems analysis is that as a procedure it is "a systematic approach to helping a decision maker choose a course of action by investigating his full problem, searching out his objectives and alternatives, using an appropriate framework—insofar as possible analytic—to bring expert judgment and intuition to bear on the problem."[8]

Program planning is considered primarily as a decision-making process. System development or system design are also terms that could be employed for the same purpose. Basic to all of these is the factor of human choice or decision-making. It is assumed that more rational choices can and will be made by the utilization of some systems analysis procedural framework, but error

[8] E. S. Quade, "Introduction," in *Systems Analysis and Policy Planning*, ed. E. S. Quade and W. I. Boucher (New York: American Elsevier Publishing Company, Inc., 1968), p. 2.

Application of Systems Analysis Procedures to Program Planning

remains feasible since the human component is the ultimate decision maker at each level.

A systems analysis program planning framework is a flexible tool and should be considered just that. No one set procedure should be viewed as totally acceptable and applicable as presented. The procedure described is meant to be comprehensive for planning in therapeutic recreation service, but it may require adaptation or elaboration before it is put to use in a setting.

Sequencing

A basic systems analysis program planning procedure has been designed for this material. It is a combination and adaptation of four methodologies presented in the literature. Procedures were selected, adapted, or redesigned for their appropriateness to therapeutic recreation service program planning situations based on the author's familiarity with problems and factors in therapeutic recreation service. The following begins with a preliminary outline of the systems analysis program planning procedure, followed by an explanation of each step, including suitable examples for therapeutic recreation service settings. A model will thus be continuously built, described, and illustrated.

Systems Analysis Program Planning Procedure—A Methodology

Outline

Stages	Description
Conceptualization and formulation	identify issues and concerns, nature of the agency, description of clients, inventory of actual and possible resources; determine the program, system purpose, specification of objectives;
Investigation	search and compile alternative methods of reaching objectives, possible substance and process of service opportunities, possible combinations of service components;
Analysis	examine feasibility and possible consequences of alternatives; construct models for comparative and illustrative purposes;
Determination	decide on a course of action, select service components, based on available information, insight, and experience;

Design	identify purpose and objectives for each service;
	determine and design the actual substance and process for each service
	construct criteria and evaluation schemes for each service;
Operations planning	determine priority of program system objectives, assign rankings to each service;
	allocate time and resources to each service;
	design schedule;
	system preparation, train staff, purchase equipment and supplies; prepare facilities;
	determine assessment of performance schedule;
Implementation	put program system into operation (installation);
	assess performance (evaluation).

Conceptualization and Formulation

A program system must start with a clear definition of its reason to be. The purpose of the program and its associated objectives are basic to the total planning operation; however, the purpose and the objectives cannot be stated until surrounding issues and concerns are identified. Thus, the planning process begins with a discussion of factors vital to the agency. Hopefully, a group of people is involved in the planning, so varying points of view, levels of knowledge and experience, and differing orientations are combined in the sharing of insight as well as ultimate decision-making.

Among the issues and concerns to be considered in the process are: (1) the nature of the agency, (2) a description of the service recipients, (3) the environmental set, and (4) an inventory of actual and possible resources.

1. Agency: examined in terms of its origin, history, current status, and future role; who has it served; who should it serve.
2. Service recipients: description of clients; realistic assessment of the nature and needs of clients; close scrutiny of societal changes as well as medical advancements affecting clients; educational and economic factors; physical, mental, and chronological features.
3. Environmental set (factors outside the agency or department that affect

Application of Systems Analysis Procedures to Program Planning

the program and its operation): other agencies serving the same clientele; the surrounding community, transportation if clients live in the immediate community; programs of other branches or departments are considerations in an institutional setting; other systems operating in the environment; i.e., education, health services, community recreation, business, government, and religious organizations.

4. Resources (although the planning process should not be initially limited by resource capacity, basic constraints on the system need to be identified early for practical, feasible planning. Hence, identification of basic resources should be undertaken): current staff; financial assets available for expenditure; facilities and equipment; possible resources that can be realistically obtained.

The purpose of the program system can then be stated. Banathy describes the nature of the purpose as follows:

> A statement of purpose will establish the nucleus around which the system should grow. In general terms the statement tells us the reason for the system's existence. This statement should also reveal some key information about the system as a whole. It should briefly tell us about the environment of the system and about some of the broad constraints under which the system is to operate.[9]

The broad general statement of purpose becomes the backbone of the planning process. Each stage of the system development should reflect the intent of the purpose. An example of such a statement appropriate for a chronic illness unit of a large medical hospital (assuming this is a separate program entity with its own staff and resources) might read:

> To provide opportunities for service recipients to gain new leisure skills and abilities, and to exercise existing recreative abilities in order to enable recreative experience within the context of nosological limitations and the confines of the unit's facilities.

A statement of purpose for a community-based recreation program for moderately mentally retarded children might be written as follows:

> To provide an opportunity for learning and practicing recreative skills to enable recreative experience which promotes the development of appropriate social behavior and roles.

Once the purpose has been determined, the objectives can be stated. The objectives refine, describe, and specify in greater detail aspects of the purpose. Concepts such as remedial, preventative, and sustaining function may appear in these statements, since objectives indicate what has to be included to meet the systems purpose. Examples of some system objectives for the first purpose stated above might be:

[9] Banathy, *Instruction Systems*, p. 32.

1. To sustain current recreative interests of service recipients through the provision of a broad spectrum of activity offerings.
2. To prevent further deterioration of affective abilities through the introduction of new activity interests that can be carried out in the unit.
3. To provide sensory-motor activities to remediate loss of physical function (range of motion, muscle atrophy, etc.).

At this point the system purpose and objectives remain general and allow for a wide range of alternative methods and procedures to lead to their accomplishment. The system purpose and objectives provide basic direction for the planning and decision-making that is to follow. These statements are referred to as the "system's (or program's) purpose and objectives"; they are not to be confused with the specific objectives developed later which are called "service objectives." The first stage of the planning process is called "Formulation and Conceptualization" and appears in Diagram VIII.

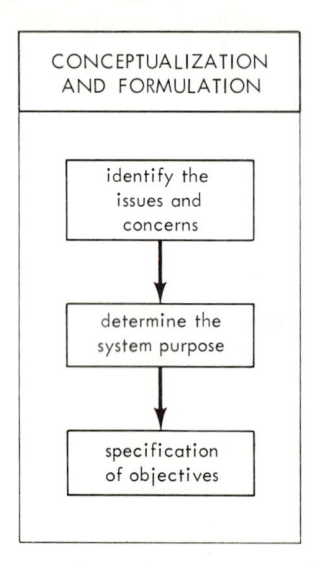

DIAGRAM VIII. CONCEPTUALIZATION AND FORMULATION

Investigation

The second stage of the planning procedure could easily be called "brainstorming," for it is at this stage that ideas are generated without regard to their eventual consequence. This process in and of itself should help to loosen existing biases of the planning group. Ideas suggested at this level become the alternatives that the decision maker later sorts through. Obviously it is to his advantage to have a wide selection of alternative methods or means to reach his objectives. For example, if one of the stated objectives has to do with teaching

Application of Systems Analysis Procedures to Program Planning

new recreative skills, a list of alternative methods of reaching this goal could appear as follows:

1. Provide equipment and facilities with self-instruction materials available;
2. Locate other clients with skills and have them teach their skills to others;
3. Select one skill area and have a staff member recruit clients for depth learning of this skill;
4. Contract for the service of specialists on a part-time basis to teach skills;
5. Use families or volunteers to teach skills;
6. Involve service recipients interested in learning with staff on a one-to-one basis;
7. Start a "skill of the month" campaign and concentrate on one activity in depth for that period;
8. Organize skill clubs and let members select teachers and recruit new client members.

Such a list could be extended with many more ideas and ways of reaching one objective. Feasibility or practicality should be played down while attempting to search out creative, innovative alternatives. It is also important not to dwell on any given idea too long or endeavor to refine or expand the idea in terms of actual operation; however, suggestions can and should be made regarding substance and process. "Investigation" is basically the process of searching and compiling alternative methods of reaching an objective or a combination of objectives.

Since this stage follows immediately after the "Conceptualization and Formulation" stage, it is diagrammed with a solid arrow indicating flow from the first stage to the second (Diagram IX).

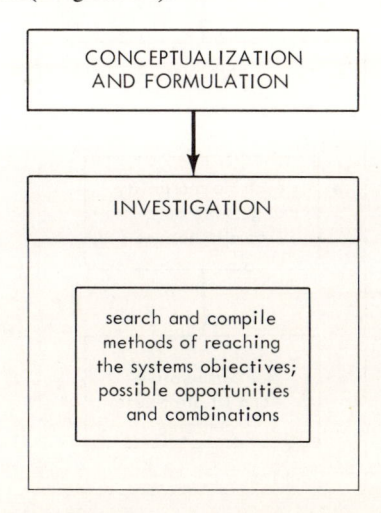

DIAGRAM IX.   INVESTIGATION

Analysis

During the "Analysis" stage, each idea suggested in the "Investigation" stage is examined in light of this feasibility, practicality, and appropriateness. An idea is explored in terms of its relationship to the purpose and the objectives of the system. Possible outcomes can be discussed as another means of predicting the value of the idea. The program matrix described previously may be utilized in the "Analysis" process, and each idea can be placed in the context of one of the twelve possible service categories. This offers the opportunity for each idea to be viewed in context of its complexity, as well as resource requirements; i.e., a service requiring leadership or teaching will require more staff time than will an administrative service (provision of supplies or equipment). Once ideas are placed in a framework of service components, models can be constructed for comparative and illustrative purposes. For example, a model may be constructed containing the best alternatives determined through the "Analysis" process. Once portrayed in model form and examined, it may be found that too many components are geared toward one objective, or too many resources are required to carry out the services depicted. The value of model building is in the comprehensive view it provides while stripping unnecessary detail and allowing

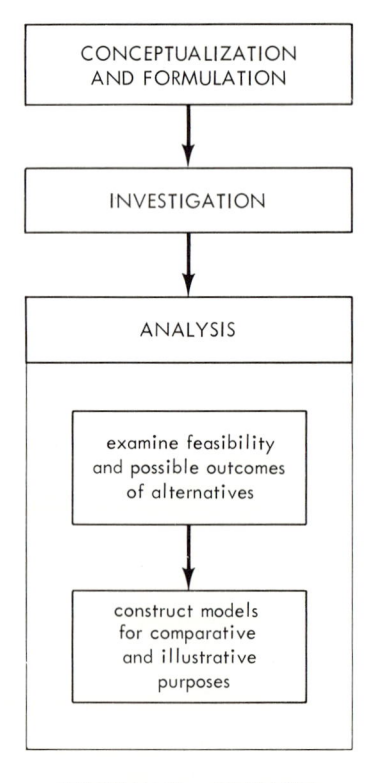

DIAGRAM X. ANALYSIS

Application of Systems Analysis Procedures to Program Planning 143

basics to be visible and compared. In planning at this level, it is important to develop a large number of models portraying possible combinations of services which might accomplish the system's goals and objectives, so decisions in the next stage can be made more realistically and with greater foresight regarding possible outcomes.

Because "Analysis" follows the "Investigation" stage, a solid arrow is used in the diagram. At this level, objectives formulated in the first stage, as well as issues and concerns of the agency, are carefully recalled and considered. Alternatives retained after "Analysis" are viable methods to obtain the system's intent (Diagram X).

Determination

Planning now requires an important decision-making step. The two previous stages have resulted in the collecting and reviewing of alternative methods of reaching the system's objectives. At this point, choices must be made by the decision maker (executive director, agency head, therapeutic recreation director, etc.) as to the course of action. Before him is the information he has available, the purpose and objectives of the system, the issues and concerns affecting his agency, and the models of the alternative means of reaching his goals. The decisions he makes reflect insight and intuition, experience, and his bias, but he makes them with a wide array of alternatives available, and with as

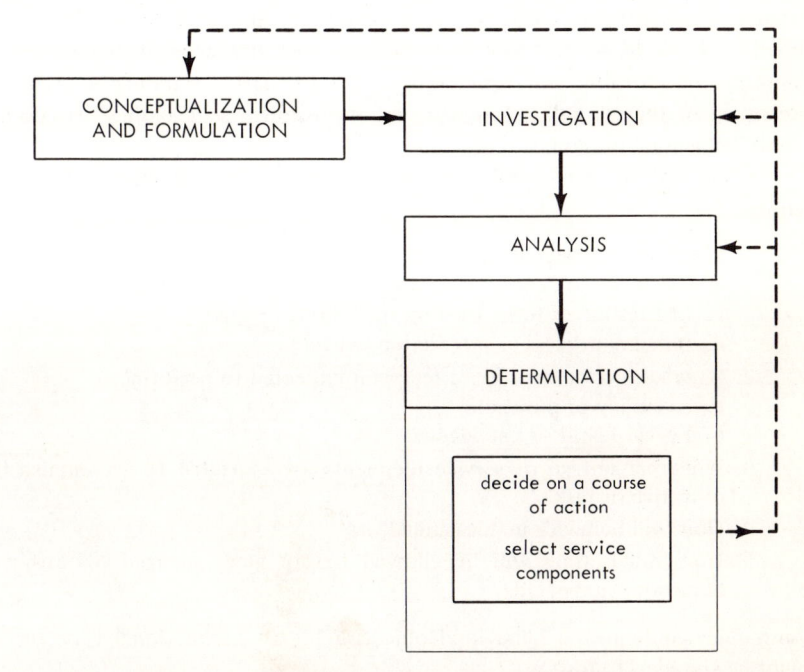

DIAGRAM XI. DETERMINATION

much information as the planning process has afforded him thus far. He selects the basic components or services for the system keeping in mind his objectives, resources, and service recipients.

Diagram XI displays a solid arrow indicating flow from stage one, through stages two and three, and into stage four, the "Determination" level in program planning. However, a feedback loop is added. If the decision maker is unable to select choices to his satisfaction, one of three routes can be taken. First, he may request that the third stage, "Analysis" be engaged again; second, he may request that the "Investigation" stage be reactivated; or third, he may decide to go back to the "Conceptualization and Formulation" stage and rewrite his purpose or objectives or both. At whatever point he re-enters the process, the methodology is reinstated at that level and continued down through the stages (Diagram XI).

Design

The decisions made in the "Determination" stage provide a "green light" for the actual design of the service components. Since the decision maker has selected the basic services he thinks will accomplish the system's objectives, his task now is to refine and develop each service. This process begins by stating the purpose and objectives for each service included. The service purpose, much like the system purpose, is stated in general terms; however, service objectives are stated very specifically. These statements are vital, since evaluation of service is directly related to service objectives. Actual, measurable behavioral outcomes comprise the wording and terminology of these latter statements. Accurate assessment of the service performance is not possible if service objectives do not specify behavioral outcomes.

When writing behavioral objectives the following guidelines may prove helpful:

1. What is the service recipient expected to do?
    a. Use verbs to denote observable behavior.
    b. List resources to be used by the service recipient.
    c. Indicate process or interaction expected.
2. At what level is the service recipient expected to perform?
    a. Accuracy or duration.
    b. Level of skill or knowledge.
3. What percentage of service recipients are expected to accomplish the objective or task?
4. How will behavior be measured?
5. How much time will be allowed before new, changed, or different behavior is expected?

Using such guidelines, a behavioral objective for an instructional type service might be stated as follows:

50 percent of the unit's population will demonstrate their ability to play a new table game of their choice, at a competitive level, with a staff member, after two months of service involvement.

Although the guidelines offered here may not be appropriate for each type of service designed, a modified form which allows for observable and measurable behavioral outcomes is a requirement. (Sources listed at the end of this chapter can assist in the preparation and writing of behavioral objectives.)

The next step in the "Design" stage is to determine the substance and process for each service component. In systems terminology this is referred to as "functions and component analysis." Having stated the purpose and behavioral objectives for each service, the task is then to design the procedure for, or method of interaction which will enable the objective to be met. This again is a decision-making process, since each objective can be accomplished through many routes or means. Decisions are made in light of other service requirements as well as available resources. Allowing all services to operate means carefully analyzing the content and processes; compromises may have to be made. If for example, a leisure counseling service is selected, its content (issues and media) must be determined as well as the interaction process to be employed. One hour per client per week may be the preferred time period, but other service components might make this optimal period impossible. The compromise of one half hour per week per client may be made, in order to continue other service requiring individual staff time, such as an instructional service.

Regardless of the shifting and changing of service component design, at the end of this period, each selected service will have an outline of the exact interaction process to be utilized, including the content, media, or substance to be employed to meet the requirements of the service objectives. If this cannot be accomplished, the planning process should revert back to a previous stage—the "Determination" stage, and thus a feedback loop appears from "Design" to "Determination" to show that another decision must be made regarding the selection of services (Diagram XII).

The final procedure in the "Design" stage is the construction of criteria tests for each service. Although the service objectives state the method of assessment, it is not an evaluation measurement. Each service requires a criteria test or performance measurement of its own. Each service may differ considerably in the form its assessment takes, or a given service may require several kinds of assessment procedures. In some cases, for example, when equipment has been placed in a lounge area, a human observer may note the frequency of use over a given time period and compare participation rates with the service objective statement. In the case of leadership service, the number of social interactions initiated by a service recipient may be part of the assessment of performance, assuming that the service objective was stated in terms of social involvement. In an instructional service, the amount of information recalled by the service recipient verbally, on paper, or a skill performance test, may comprise the evaluation. *At no point does the evaluation seek to determine whether recreative experiences are taking place.* Evaluation or criteria tests can only measure the frequency, duration, nature, or level of behavior. Whether someone has experienced recreation while engaging in an activity cannot be measured—only reported, since what has occured is a subjective psychic phenomenon.

If criteria tests or assessment measurements are impossible to construct, it may be that the objectives of a given service are improperly conceived or stated, or that the design of the substance and process are faulty. Consequently a feedback loop must also be placed between the construction of criteria

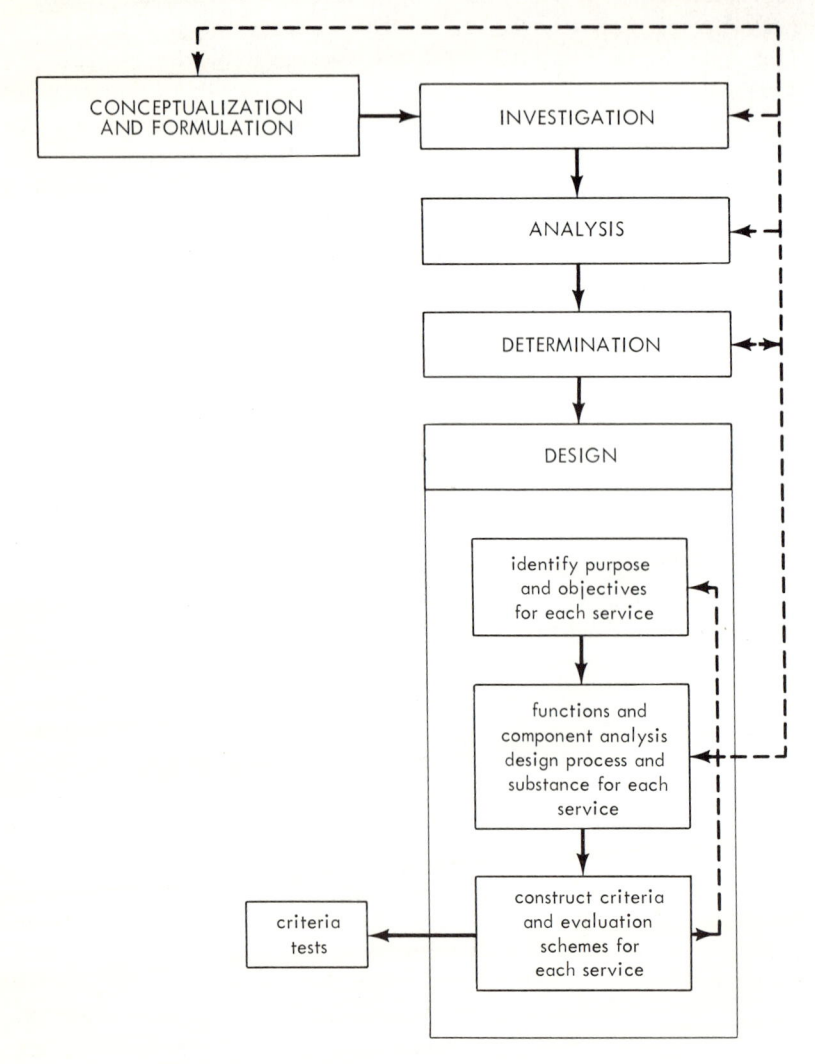

DIAGRAM XII. DESIGN

Application of Systems Analysis Procedures to Program Planning

measurement and the statement of service objectives and the design of service content and procedures. Diagram XII illustrates the criteria measurement tests as a separate unit since there will be a flow through this unit later which does not necessarily pass through the "Design" stage.

Operations Planning

This stage of the planning and decision-making procedure begins with a survey of the system's objectives. A priority or hierarchy is determined. Services associated with each objective are then given rankings. Time and resources can then be distributed or allocated to each service. Although service components have been designed in the previous stage, a determination is not made until this stage. *How much* or *how often* a service will be employed must be decided upon at this stage. If services have been misjudged in terms of complexity or resource use, planning reverts back to one of two stages; i.e., the "Design" stage may be reactivated and the service simplified, or the "Determination" stage may be

```
          ↓
    ┌─────────────────┐
    │  DETERMINATION  │◄─ ─ ┐
    └─────────────────┘     │
          ↓                 │
    ┌─────────────────┐     │
    │     DESIGN      │◄─ ┐ │
    └─────────────────┘   │ │
          ↓               │ │
┌─────────────────────────┴─┴───┐
│    OPERATIONS PLANNING        │
│  ┌─────────────────────────┐  │
│  │ priority of objectives  │  │
│  │ ranking of service      │──┘
│  │ distribution of resources│
│  │   and time              │
│  │ design schedule         │
│  └─────────────────────────┘
│          ↓
│  ┌─────────────────────────┐
│  │   system preparation    │
│  └─────────────────────────┘
│          ↓
│  ┌─────────────────────────┐
│  │ assessment of performance│
│  │       schedule           │
│  └─────────────────────────┘
└───────────────────────────────┘
```

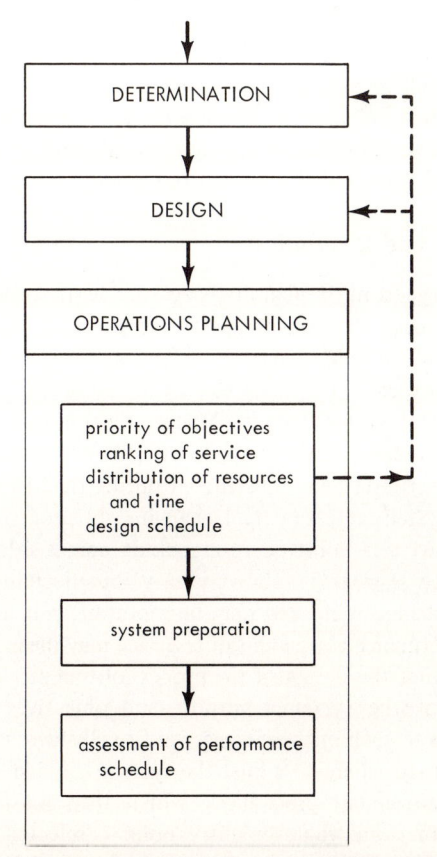

DIAGRAM XIII. OPERATIONS PLANNING

re-entered and a decision made to remove a service—hence the feedback loops to these two prior stages.

After the schedule has been developed, system preparation begins. This procedure can be lengthy, depending on the size, auspices, or type of setting involved. For example, in a new program, personnel may need to be hired as well as trained. This step also includes a variety of administrative tasks such as the ordering of equipment and supplies, readiness of the facilities, establishing report and record routines, and a variety of other tasks required for actual operation of the system. Considerable time will be spent in staff training since many individuals are not acquainted with "management by objectives" programs. Resistance can run high, due to a lack of understanding of the concepts, and because of the staff's expectations. This may be alleviated by adequate orientation and training sessions. Training is also vital since more exact interaction patterns and processes are designed into the service components. Accurate assessment of the systems performance requires that there be stability and reliability in the processes used to reach the stated objectives.

The final step in the "Operations Planning" stage is the establishment of an assessment of performance schedule. This means deciding when and how often the system will be assessed and adjusted. For example, it may be decided that each service will be assessed two months after installation, or that certain services will be assessed at different frequencies with comprehensive review in six months. A cut-away model of this stage is presented in Diagram XIII.

Implementation and Evaluation

The final stage is not a planning stage per se; it is the verification of the total planning process and the system's operation. A therapeutic recreation program system, unlike other systems which can be quantified and tested by computer simulation, can only be assessed by actual operation.

After the "Operations Planning" stage, the program system is installed. According to the predetermined schedule, its performance is measured at some point utilizing the criteria tests constructed during the "Design" stage. The step which follows is system adjustment of changing the program system to improve its performance. At this point decision-making comes into play. Determining where performance is weak is relatively easy, but deciding at what stage the improvement or change is needed may be more difficult. For example, a poor evaluation or performance assessment of a service may mean that a criteria test is inappropriate, or that the design of the process of that service was weak, or that the formulation of the system's purpose and objectives are faulty. Thus a feedback loop goes to each of these stages, and to all stages inbetween.

A decision as to where to adjust the system is made, and is accompanied by associated improvement procedures, which then must be followed down through the system from whatever entry point is selected. The process of the system's operation is one of continual evaluation and adjustment. The program system may never be completely optimized, although definite improvements can

Application of Systems Analysis Procedures to Program Planning 149

be made. Thus planning and decision-making remain active, since the program system will continue to be cyclical. The completed model of the systems analysis program planning procedure appears in Diagram XIV.

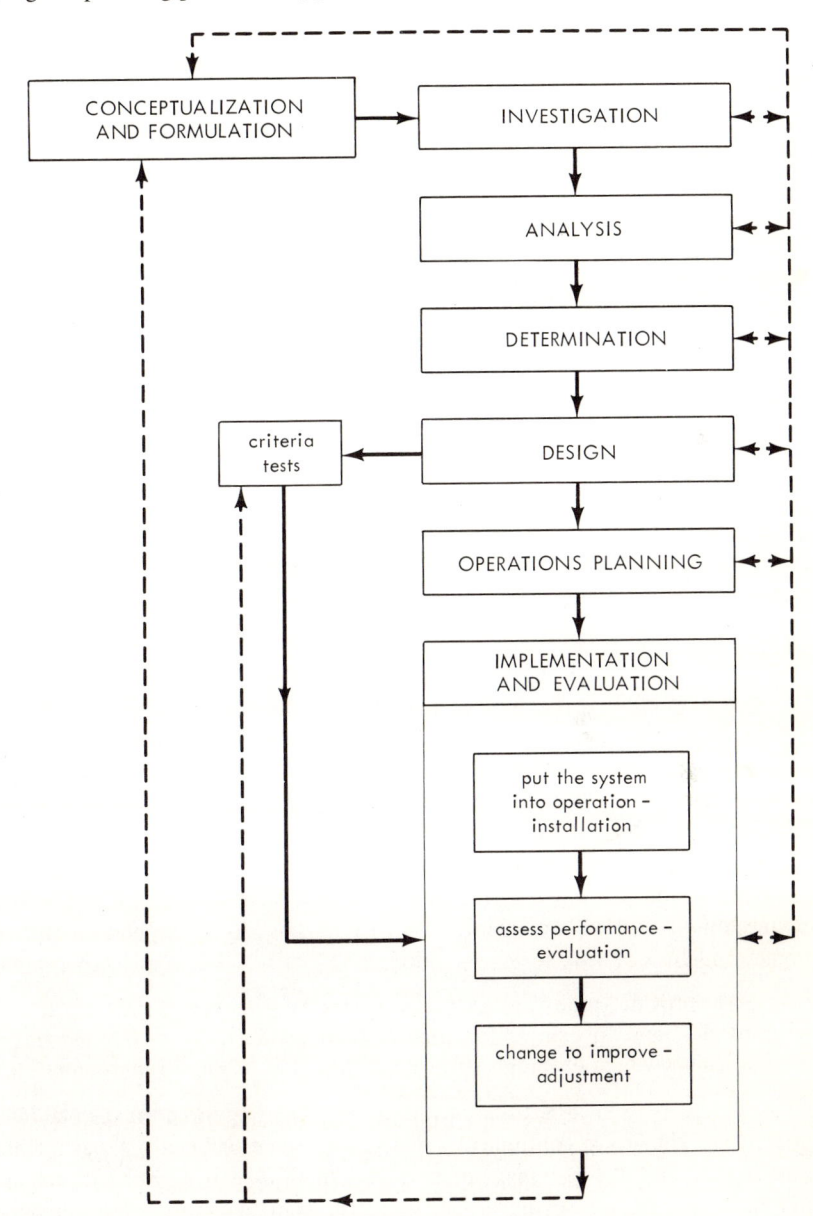

DIAGRAM XIV.   IMPLEMENTATION, EVALUATION AND COMPLETED SYSTEMS ANALYSIS PROGRAM PLANNING MODEL

Application of the Procedure

For the purpose of illustrating the application of the systems analysis program planning procedure, a hypothetical setting and population will be presented. A nursing home with a capacity of sixty comprises the arbitrarily selected group. It will be assumed that two-thirds of the residents are ambulatory and require minimum nursing care and attention. The other third are in an infirmary or extended care program. The therapeutic recreation program is to serve both groups of residents. One full time therapeutic recreation specialist, and one full-time paraprofessional comprise the staff. In addition, some nursing time will be allotted to the recreation program. Involved in the initial stages of planning will be the therapeutic recreation staff, an outside therapeutic recreation consultant, the director of the home, a member of the nursing staff, and possibly a social service staff member.

Conceptualization and Formulation

The planning team begins with a discussion of the nature of the agency itself. Its sponsorship, organization, purposes, issues confronting their current operations, its historical origins, and new directions in service may be among the concerns presented. Second, they discuss the nature of the residents of the home. Factors such as age, ethnic and occupational background, physical and mental conditions, etc. are examined. This is followed by an inventory of actual and possible resources. The nature of the facility itself, community resources, volunteer potential, financial considerations, expansion possibilities, etc. are brought into the conversation. Next, environmental issues are discussed. Other agencies and organizations influencing their operation, governmental regulations, medical and health standards, trends in nursing home operation, etc. are identified. This preliminary discussion level allows the planning team to take a solid look at its agency and residents before actual design of the program. Issues and concerns raised here are used continously as the planning proceeds from stage to stage.

Next the group determines the therapeutic recreation program purpose and develops a written statement. For this nursing home population such a statement might read as follows:

> To provide opportunities for residents to gain new leisure skills and attitudes, and to exercise existing recreative abilities to enable recreative experience which promotes social, cognitive, and physical functioning.

This statement then becomes the backbone and directing force for the planning that follows. The group continues by developing specific objectives that further refine and expand the statement of purpose. These objectives will indicate the function of service, yet remain broad. From the statement above, the following objectives for this nursing home recreation program are:

1. To sustain current recreative interests of the residents through provision of a broad range of activity offerings.

Application of Systems Analysis Procedures to Program Planning 151

   2. To prevent cognitive and sensory motor impairment by introducing new recreative activities and opportunities.
   3. To prevent and remediate social isolation through provision of interaction oriented activities.
   4. To develop appropriate leisure attitudes through counseling and activity involvement.

The above objectives indicate direction, but not exact content or definite structure of the services to be offered.

Investigation

The second stage is one of suggesting ways of meeting the developed objectives. Ideas are presented as in a "brainstorming" session. All suggestions are placed on a list for later analysis. The goal at this point is to loosen thinking and come up with a wide variety of ideas related to each of the objectives. A list of ideas related to the *third* objective might read as follows:

   1. Have an orientation for each new resident regarding the purpose of the program and the nature of resident involvement;
   2. Provide a host or hostess at one meal a day to promote interaction;
   3. Stress interaction during activities through leadership involvement in activity offerings;
   4. Counsel residents regarding need for social involvement;
   5. Present group-oriented service projects;
   6. Introduce a resident a week on a bulletin board;
   7. Provide family recreation nights at the home;
   8. Teach only skills that require interaction between two or more people;
   9. Have a cocktail hour before the evening meal;
   10. Organize small clubs around interest areas.

A similar list would be developed for each of the written objectives.

Analysis

At this stage, each of the ideas presented in the "Investigation" stage would be analyzed for their possibilities and potential. Issues and concerns, the statement of purpose and the objectives are kept in mind while examining each idea.

Some of the investigated ideas suggested for the *third* objective might come through this process in the following manner:

   a. Ideas No. 1 and 4 be combined;
   b. Idea No. 2 changed to two meals per week, because of staffing problems;
   c. Idea No. 3 combined with ideas suggested for objective *one*;
   d. Idea No. 7 dropped due to too few residents with families in the immediate vicinity.

Some ideas would be expanded and tangents explored, others would be modified, some dropped. Possible outcomes related to each alternative would be discussed. At the conclusion of this stage, a list of feasible alternatives, plus models of possible combinations will have been developed.

Determination

The planning group or a predetermined member now selects a course of action by choosing from the alternatives presented. This decision is made in light of all information available, plus experience, insight, and intuition. A wide array of possible alternatives and their predicted outcomes helps to make rational selections of service components.

Design

At this stage, the planning group is reduced to those individuals who are most capable of designing the actual therapeutic recreation program. In this case, the individuals concerned are the therapeutic recreation specialist and the consultant. Each service will be designed and developed. Included in this step will be the determination of the purpose, the establishment of behavioral objectives, the design of the substance, process or interaction technique, and the development of criteria tests for each service.

Assume that an education-preventative component has been selected related to the social isolation and leisure counseling objectives. The purpose of the service might read as follows:

> To prevent social isolation of the resident through individual counseling which focuses on information sharing and attitude development.

One of the behavioral objectives of this service might be:

> 50 percent of the ambulatory residents (infirmary excluded) will verbally recall the names of ten other residents and relate one fact about the background of each of those individuals, after three months of service involvement.

The process of the education-preventative service could be described as follows:

1. Each new resident will be interviewed by the therapeutic recreation specialist shortly after arrival (2 to 5 days);
2. Thereafter, the resident will be "visited" and counseled for one half hour once every two weeks;
3. Interaction will stress informal *dialogue*

The content or substance of the counseling sessions could be described as follows:

1. Information related to the recreation service of the home and opportunities for social interaction;

Application of Systems Analysis Procedures to Program Planning 153

    2. Information related to the nature of social isolation and its results;
    3. Expectations of the home related to the resident's responsibility to self and others regarding social involvement;
    4. Development of a positive attitude toward time and the opportunities it offers for self-satisfaction and fulfillment.

One of the criteria tests for this service would include a verbal question and answer period. The therapeutic recreation specialist after three months would ask the resident to tell him about some of the people he has met at the home. (This method is in keeping with the informal dialogue interaction process established.) The therapeutic recreation specialist would, however, note the number of names and facts recalled and probe if necessary ("Is there anyone else you have gotten to know since coming here?").

The entire procedure of establishment of purpose, behavioral objectives, process and substance (or content), and criteria tests would be developed for each service component in this "Design" stage.

Operations Planning

"Operations Planning" involves a variety of steps necessary prior to actual program implementation. First, the decision maker decides on the priority of the system's objectives. In this case, he may have decided that the "socialization" objective was first, followed in order by the "teaching of new skills," "leisure attitudes," and last, the "exercising of existing recreative abilities" objective. Each of the service components are then ranked to correspond with the objective hierarchy. Once these decisions are made, allocation of time and resources follows. Since this is a small operation, services may have been developed with staff considerations taken into account during the "Design" stage. Length and frequency of services are determined and a schedule of the system program is developed. For the nursing-home program this would probably be in the form of a weekly schedule with service components and staff blocked in.

Next would be system preparation. This level includes a variety of administrative tasks, such as the purchase of equipment and supplies, facilities preparation; training of the paraprofessional, volunteers, and the nursing staff assigned to the program. Record and reporting procedures are developed. Additional tasks might include a presentation to the Board of Directors, some public relations work with families, and resident readiness.

The final step in "Operations Planning" is the determination of when the system will be evaluated and adjusted. With a new program in a nursing home, the program should probably operate at least two months before evaluations, since many factors outside the actual system design may influence the output of the program. Minor adjustments may be made during these early weeks regarding time scheduling, but major changes in services should wait until a complete assessment can be made. The assessment schedule will also be influenced by the actual wording of the behavioral objectives of each service. If the objective states that three months will be allowed for the development of a specific behavior, then that aspect of the system should not be evaluated prior to that time.

Implementation and Evaluation

The final stage of the planning procedure is the actual implementation of the program. At this point the various service components are put into operation with the residents of the home and allowed to operate for the previously established period of time.

Assessment of the system's performance follows. Each service component is evaluated according to the criteria tests developed in the "Design" stage. The results of the assessment will indicate problem areas, and adjustments can be made. Entire services may be omitted, or changed, criteria tests may be re-examined for their value, changes in process or interaction methods may be altered, behavioral objectives may be rewritten. It is probable that the consultant would be called in to aid in the assessment, evaluation, and system adjustment process. His opinion as to system performance in addition to staff and resident input would allow for more objective assessment and consequent system improvement. The nursing-home program would then continue to operate with the adjustments made. Thus the operation, assessment, and adjustment cycle continues as long as the therapeutic recreation program exists.

Sources for Preparing and Writing Behavioral Objectives

Armstrong, Robert J., Terry D. Cornell, Robert E. Kraner, and E. Wayne Roberson, *The Development and Evaluation of Behavioral Objectives.* Worthington, Ohio: Charles A. Jones Publishing Company, 1970.

Gagné, Robert M., *The Conditions of Learning.* New York: Holt, Rinehart and Winston, 1965.

——. "Educational Objectives and Human Performance," in *Learning and the Educational Process,* ed. J. D. Krumboltz. Chicago: Rand McNally, 1965.

Gronlund, Norman E., *Stating Behavioral Objectives for Classroom Instruction.* London: The Macmillan Company, 1970.

Hitch, C. J., "On the Choice of Objectives in Systems Studies," in *Systems Research and Design,* ed. Donald P. Eckman. New York: John Wiley and Sons, Inc., 1961.

Mager, Robert F., *Preparing Instructional Objectives.* Palo Alto, California: Fearon Publishers, 1962.

Smith, Robert G., Jr., *The Design of Instructional Systems,* Technical Report 66-18. Alexandria, Va.: Hum RRO, 1966.

——. *The Development of Training Objectives,* Research Bulletin 11. Alexandria, Va.: Hum RRO, 1964.

Tyler, Ralph W., "Some Persistent Questions on the Defining of Objectives," in *Defining Educational Objectives,* ed. C. M. Lindvall. Pittsburgh: University of Pittsburgh Press, 1964.

10
Social and Behavioral Factors in Program Organization

There are many techniques that can be utilized in organizing a therapeutic recreation program. Each of the elements of service (see Chapters 6 and 7) may be offered through a number of organizational structures. For example, in order to stimulate the improvement of general health and appearance, a recreation specialist may hold an individual conference with a patient or client in his office, or he may involve the patient or client in a formal grooming class; he may make informal comments and suggestions to the patient or client during a lounge program, or he may invite the patient or client to view a motion picture on the subject and then to participate in a lecture/discussion; he may manipulate peer pressure at a club meeting, or he may use some other structure.

From these few examples concerning one element of service, it is apparent that the key factors to consider in program organization are (1) how the specialist will use himself, (2) what type of structure and interactive process he will employ, and (3) which substantive content will be selected as the medium for action. This chapter offers information regarding these three aspects of program organization drawing upon information from the behavioral and social sciences.

Leadership Roles

Regardless of the assigned level of responsibility, all persons who lead others play one or more social roles during the course of an activity. A role is a function taken or assumed by someone. Each role has a status

Social and Behavioral Factors in Program Organization 157

or social position that indicates how much authority or power over others an individual possesses. Any leadership role may be superimposed on an activity. A number of roles may be used interchangeably during an activity, or a single role may be played throughout the duration of an activity. One role may be used consistently throughout the duration of a number of activities over a relatively long period of time. A specialist selects a role based upon the patient or client's *relative level of maturity*—that is, *how much internal control over his own behavior a patient or client manifests,* and *how much external control is needed in order to function effectively in social situations.*

In the following, eight leadership roles are presented with examples of leader behavior and status. These are pure types, and require considerable experience for someone to play consistently. These roles should be viewed as a horizontal continuum rather than in a vertical hierarchy. More than likely, a specialist will select aspects of each role and incorporate these aspects as part of his unique leadership style, based upon his own level of personal development and integration. A horizontal conceptualization permits one to move back and forth between roles with relative ease. Rapid role modifications are made in relation to patient or client situational needs or as a consequence of immediate behavioral changes during activity involvement.

CONTROLLER

The Controller makes all decisions regarding action. He decides what activity will be engaged in, who will engage in it, for what period of time, and in which place. He checks and regulates participant involvement in the activity. He sets the rules, sees that they are followed, and defines the limits in which the participant may operate. He exercises restraining power over participants, and dominates the situation.

It is obvious from this description that the role lends itself to situations in which patients or clients have little internal control and a considerable degree of external control must be exercised. This role is often played with small children and with adolescents and adults who are hyperactive or who are not responsible for their behavior. It is also played with persons who have difficulty in making decisions as a consequence of illness, and at times is used in operant conditioning programs with the mentally retarded child. Sometimes an activity may pose a hazard to certain patients or clients and this role is utilized to permit continued participation.

DIRECTOR

The Director actively leads, but does not make all the decisions. He allows the participant some personal latitude. The Director decides where, when, how, and who concerning action. He causes participants to follow a specific course of action. He points out the right way to act. He regulates the action and the course of this action. He gives orders or instructions in an authoritative manner. He commands, manages, guides the selection of behavioral effects to be produced, and the means to be used. He indicates the appropriate tempo, mood, and intensity of the action.

Although in this role some degree of internal participant control is assumed, the participant has need to know all of the limits of action in order to behave effectively. He relies on the leader to set these limits. This role is often played with children and adults who are mentally ill, and at times with others who as a result of disability are relearning to live within the scope of an altered life situation. The role is sometimes played in correctional institutions with persons who manifest asocial behavior.

INSTIGATOR

The Instigator starts action, gets participants involved, and then moves out of a direct leadership role. He sets minimal limits and expects some degree of participant control. He respects individuality and encourages expressions of self-determination. He goads and urges participants to act. He provokes and incites them, getting them to move forward.

This role is used with persons who are lethargic, depressed, bored, spiritless, indifferent, preoccupied, and apathetic. The intent is to get them involved. As an Instigator, the leader may wish to have a participant become actively involved to express real feelings—feelings that may be negative. For example, in a communal living situation for the elderly, a client may be quite angry that he is there, but may be unable to say so. As a consequence, the client bottles up angry feelings and thus begins to suffer a number of uncomfortable physical symptoms. It may be the specialist's function (using this role) to provoke the client into expressing his anger. In a psychiatric setting, a patient may consistently reject certain negative ideas about his behavior during psychotherapeutic interviews by indicating that he never behaves in a specific manner. A psychiatrist may request that the specialist play the role of instigator, inciting certain behavior in the patient so the patient may be presented with tangible evidence that he does indeed behave in the ways he has denied. This latter task is especially difficult and requires considerable supervision and experience.

STIMULATOR

The Stimulator generates positive interest in activity and stands by to encourage and assist participation when necessary. He excites, stirs, impels, and rouses participants.

This role is often used in work with mentally retarded young persons, also those with physical disability who are relearning patterns of behavior, and at times with elderly persons in nursing homes and related facilities.

EDUCATOR

The Educator teaches skills which the participant wishes to learn so that he may become more active and more socially involved. The leader not only teaches activity skill per se, but is concerned with the conduct of self and effective social behavior.

This role is played in a number of settings. It assumes that a participant is self-determining and requests direct help from the leader. The role is sometimes played by a special volunteer who has a degree of expertise with specific activity media.

ADVISER

The Adviser makes suggestions to participants concerning involvement and behavior. He also makes recommendations regarding decisions or courses of action. He may counsel or give guidance and information.

This role may be played with persons in a correctional setting, or with mentally ill persons during the predischarge period. It may also be played with patients or clients in congregate living situations who have difficulty in social situations, or with persons who have a degree of physical disability and are endeavoring to take their place in society once again.

OBSERVER

The Observer watches the participant as he engages in activity. He takes notice of behavior, and recognizes the underlying meaning of various actions. He considers the meaning of what the participant does, and marks *attentively* what is happening. He perceives, evaluates, and makes *appropriate* responses to expressions of attitudes and feelings.

In this role, the leader is primarily offering sanction and realistic response by his physical presence at an activity and by what he says to the participant. It is a time when the participant is testing his wings and seeks a referent to determine his effectiveness. The role may be played in any number of settings as a consequence of treatment termination. In effect, in this role the leader is the good parent, or the "fan." However, the leader playing this role goes beyond observation in a physical sense by responding appropriately to the participant's request for response—be it approbation, critique, or chastisement.

ENABLER

The Enabler assists the participant when asked. He provides the kind of assistance the participant wishes when the participant wishes it. He gives strength or authority to the participant's purpose, and makes practicable or easy his action. He provides means and opportunities for the participant to engage in the activity of the participant's choice. The leader enhances the self-esteem and self-determination of the participant.

This role is predicated upon the fact that the patient or client is a mature person with considerable control over his life. The leader is there to make it possible for the patient or client to do what he wants to do. This role is often played in congregate living facilities and community agencies in which potential participants can and do make their own judgments and decisions regarding program content. The role may also be played in a general hospital with patients who are in a "self-care" stage and are in the process of recuperating from a short-term illness.

Structure and Interactive Process

In reality all individual patients or clients who receive therapeutic recreation service are part of what might be considered a "collection of individuals." This collection of individuals is often thought of as the patient or client "group." Popularly, any collection of individuals, whether in a classroom, on a ward, or in a stadium, are often referred to as a "group." For our purposes, a "group" has specific interactive meaning and does not mean just a "collection of individuals."

Interactive structures can be described in different ways. In recreation service in general, we describe program structures in organizational terms; that is, interviews, informal groupings, clubs, classes, interest groups, leagues, tournaments, contests, special events, mass activities, and the like. In therapeutic recreation service, it is also necessary to understand interactive processes that can be superimposed upon organizational structures—processes that affect behavior. The following selected information from the field of group dynamics indicates aspects that are applicable to therapeutic recreation service.

STRUCTURES

Service elements can be organized into an *informal lounge program;* that is, a large multipurpose area open to patients or clients for drop-in purposes. A range of simultaneous activities can be offered at this time within this setting. A card game may be going on in one part of the room while some patients or clients engage in sewing and weaving in another part of the room. Others may just sit and chat, and still others may meet with a staff member over a cup of coffee. Activity in a lounge program is primarily self-directed by participants. Staff provides sanction, some instruction, and informal guidance and counseling.

This type of structure is helpful in each program, for it offers an opportunity for patients and clients to be self-directing. In effect, such a setting takes the place of the living room or family room within the home environment of the patient or client. It is a place to which a patient or client can bring visitors so they may interact in a social manner around a pleasant experience, rather than having visitors spend the time asking the patient or client how he feels and how he is being cared for. It is also a place where patients or clients can view staff in different roles. This latter aspect enhances inmate-staff relationships.

A lounge program may function as a first step toward getting a patient or client into more structured aspects of the program, or it may act as a terminal phase of the program, offering less structure to someone preparing for discharge. Finally, because of the lack of apparent structure, it permits a patient or client to be himself and thus the situation lends itself to observation of behavior for diagnostic and evaluative purposes.

Service elements can also be organized into formal organizational patterns which foster meetings of numbers of patients or clients with a specialist on a regularly scheduled basis. The first of these formal patterns would be a *club*. A club has a membership who have some special identity signifying that they are members of a select group. A club offers patients and clients who are members a unique status and a sense of individuality. The specialist may completely sponsor a club, partially sponsor a club, or the members may develop a club on their own. The specialist who completely sponsors a club would supply the leadership and necessary equipment, schedule the time, and indicate the meeting place, while partial sponsorship may mean only some organizing help, some guidance when requested, and the selection of a meeting place. If the members organize their own club, they may require only a meeting place, or perhaps only some stimulation and sanction.

Another way to organize service elements is in formal *classes*. Classes are scheduled and structured by the specialist, who endeavors to teach specific knowledges and skills to a specified group. He may enlist the aid of volunteers to teach special skills. A class has a regular, specified membership. Patients or clients elect to join certain classes or they may be required to take certain classes as part of the care plan.

A third organizational pattern would be that of special *interest groups*. These would be scheduled activity sessions for aggregates of patients or clients who have a common interest in an activity. Time would be spent engaging in the activity, learning more about it, and making plans concerning the activity. Usually the most knowledgeable and skilled person in the group would offer leadership. The same persons might not attend the special interest group consistently, and some persons may prefer this to the more formally organized clubs or classes. A *committee* is a form of special interest group which usually has a small consistent membership and a short life, dependent upon the assigned task.

Leagues, tournaments. and *contests* are a fourth way to organize elements of service. In these organizational patterns, skilled patients or clients are selected to participate in activity on a competitive basis. Activity is organized and directed by the specialist.

Special events are yet another means of organizing activity. This might be a series of activities around a theme such as a religious holiday or civic celebration, or an agency open house, or the season of the year. The specialist involves certain patients or clients in this series of activities, which he plans and directs. Special events might also include trips to activity sessions away from the place of sponsorship, such as a theater party, a trip to the race track, or dining out in a restaurant.

A final way of organizing program would be in *mass activity* such as motion-picture viewing, parties, concerts, and the like. In these activities, the specialist organizes and conducts activities for all patients or clients who wish to attend.

In addition to these "group" structures, there are the dyadic structures in which some elements of service can be offered. A dyad is an interactive relationship between two people. The relationship can be abstracted and distinguished from other relationships so it can be considered an entity in itself. A dyad may consist of a recreation specialist and a patient or client, or a volunteer and a patient or client. The dyad is formed to accomplish a specific purpose. The substance of the interaction between the members of the dyad is often an interview; however, it may involve nonverbal interactive behavior.

Interviews can be classified into three types: (1) the *initial interview* between the patient or client and the specialist during the early stages of service is held to assess interest and needs or to help the patient or client enter into the activity program, or for other evaluation or diagnostic purposes; (2) *casual interviews* occur when a patient or client seeks personal help from the specialist or wishes assistance during a group activity session; (3) *scheduled interviews* are for counseling purposes, educational purposes, or other activity purposes. This latter aspect may be conducted in the specialist's office or in a residential institution in the room of a patient or client. A volunteer may be used in a dyadic relationship during activity programming when a patient or client is not ambulatory and cannot come to a regular activity session, or when a patient or client cannot tolerate a relationship with more than one person at a time, or when there is a special skill to be taught to an individual patient or client.

INTERACTIVE PROCESS

Within each of the organizational patterns, certain interactive processes are inherent or can be superimposed. The interactive process limits, influences, or regulates the behavior of persons engaged in the process. There are eight interactive processes identifiable at this time. Each pattern appears to be a normal means of interacting at different stages of life. Apparently one masters a pattern, includes it in his behavioral repertoire, and then attempts to master another pattern. The patterns may be developmental in nature: that is, there may be a sequence involving mastery—one must learn a specific pattern and master it before attempting to meet with success in a subsequent pattern. Affective impairment seems to foster regression to patterns mastered early in life. It has also been theorized that attempts to cope by an adult who *supposedly* has mastered all of the interaction patterns sometimes fosters affective impairment if true mastery does not exist.

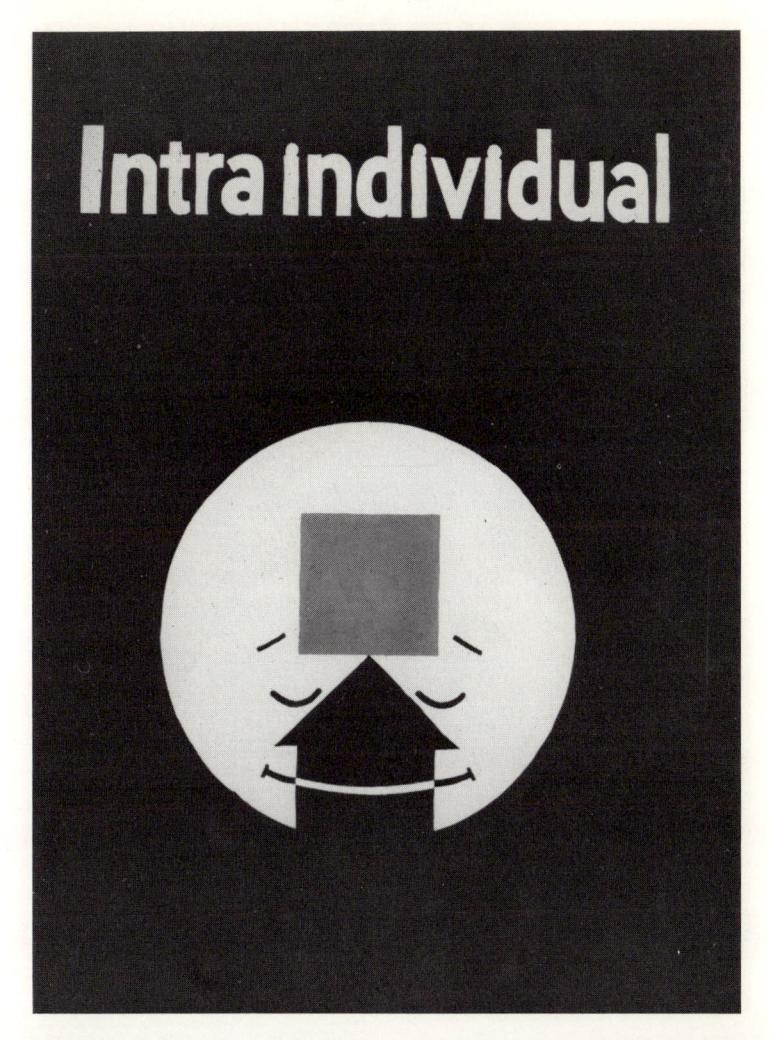

PROCESS I. INTRA-INDIVIDUAL

Action taking place within the mind of a person or action involving the mind and a part of the body, but requiring no contact with another person or external object. This type of interaction is characteristic of normal infants, adults who are severely psychotic, and adults engaged in daydreaming. It is not a pattern that one would superimpose on an organizational structure, but may be a starting place when working with some patients or clients who are "loners." (See Figure 1.)

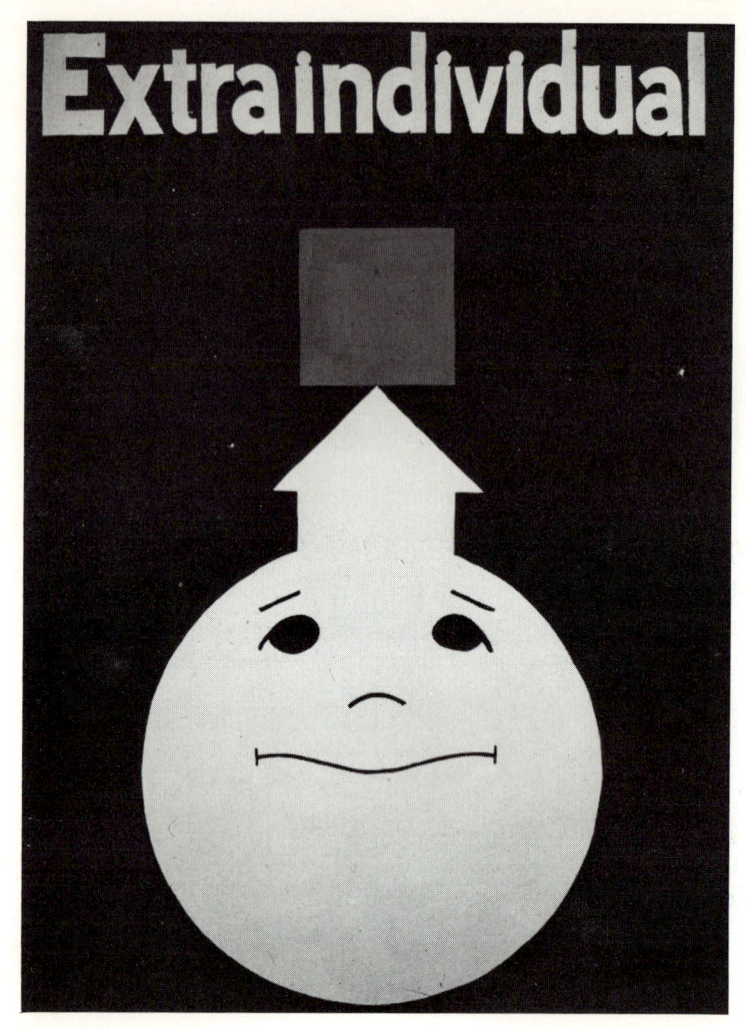

PROCESS II. EXTRA-INDIVIDUAL

Action directed by a person toward an object in the environment, requiring no contact with another person. This process is inherent in reading, walking, most solitary art or craft activity, viewing television alone, and so forth. It is characteristic of children with short attention spans, some adults who are psychotic, and also severely retarded persons. (See Figure 2.)

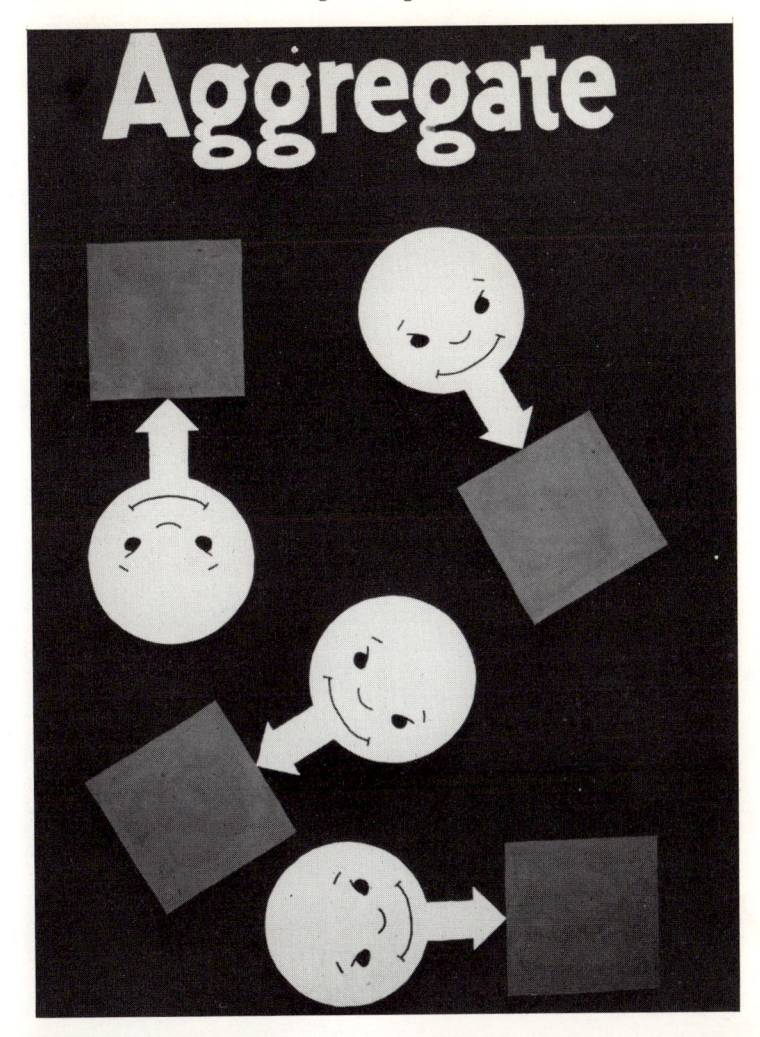

Social and Behavioral Factors in Program Organization 165

PROCESS III. AGGREGATE

Action directed by a person toward an object in the environment while in the company of other persons who are also directing action toward objects in the environment. Action is not directed toward one another, and no interaction between participants is required or necessary. This process is inherent in motion-picture viewing, watching a play, in a bingo game, in a craft shop, and so forth. It is what the literature refers to as parallel play in small children. It is a process a specialist may use as the first step toward fostering interaction at a higher level. (See Figure 3.)

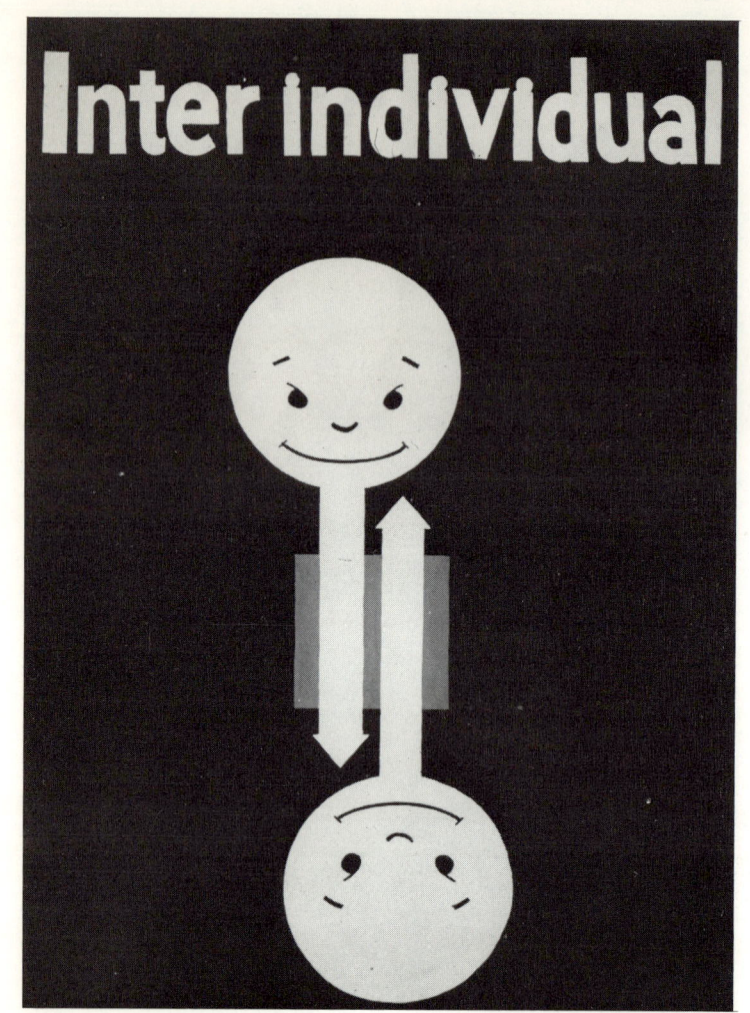

PROCESS IV. INTER-INDIVIDUAL

Action of a competitive nature directed by one person toward another. This is the first of the true dyadic relationships. It is inherent in chess, checkers, and a variety of other two-person encounters. Because the interaction is competitive, a specialist would not seek to use this process in interview sessions. Unfortunately some persons view all dyadic relationships as inter-individual, and as a consequence, cannot enter into a close relationship with one other person, e.g.—supervision, friendship, marriage. (See Figure 4.)

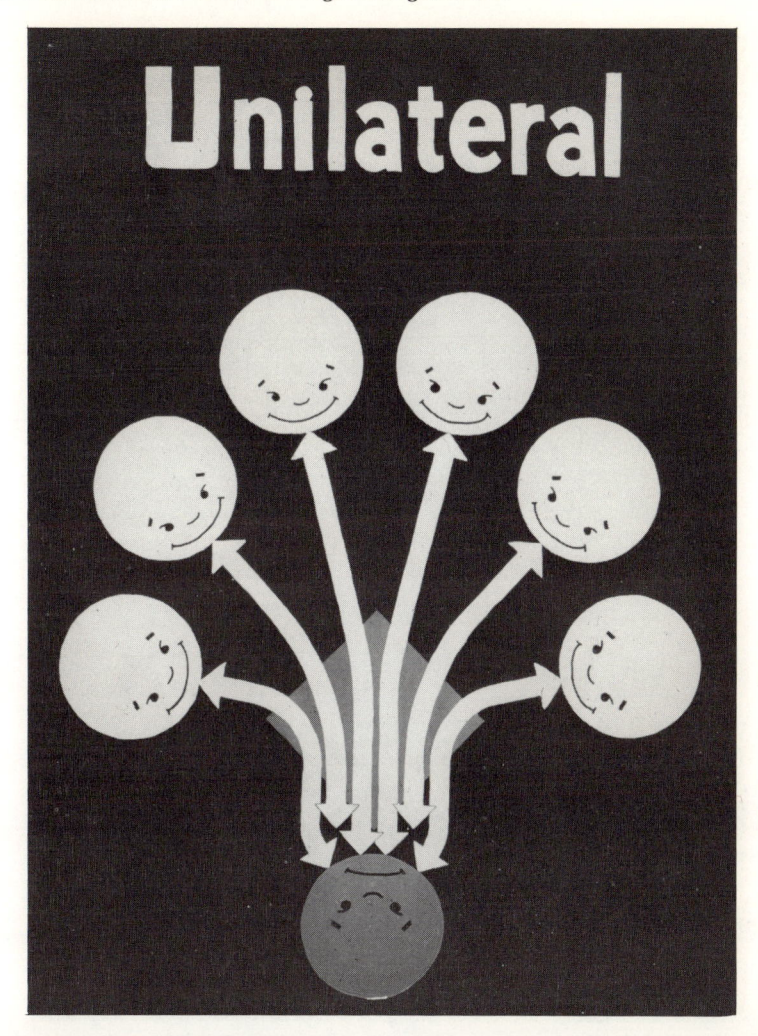

Social and Behavioral Factors in Program Organization   167

PROCESS V. UNILATERAL

Action of a competitive nature among three or more persons, one of whom is an antagonist or *it*. Interaction is in simultaneous competitive dyadic relationships. Although this pattern may be characteristic of young children, it often can be found in adult congregate living situations, and in an activity situation in which participants are vying for the leader's attention. (See Figure 5.)

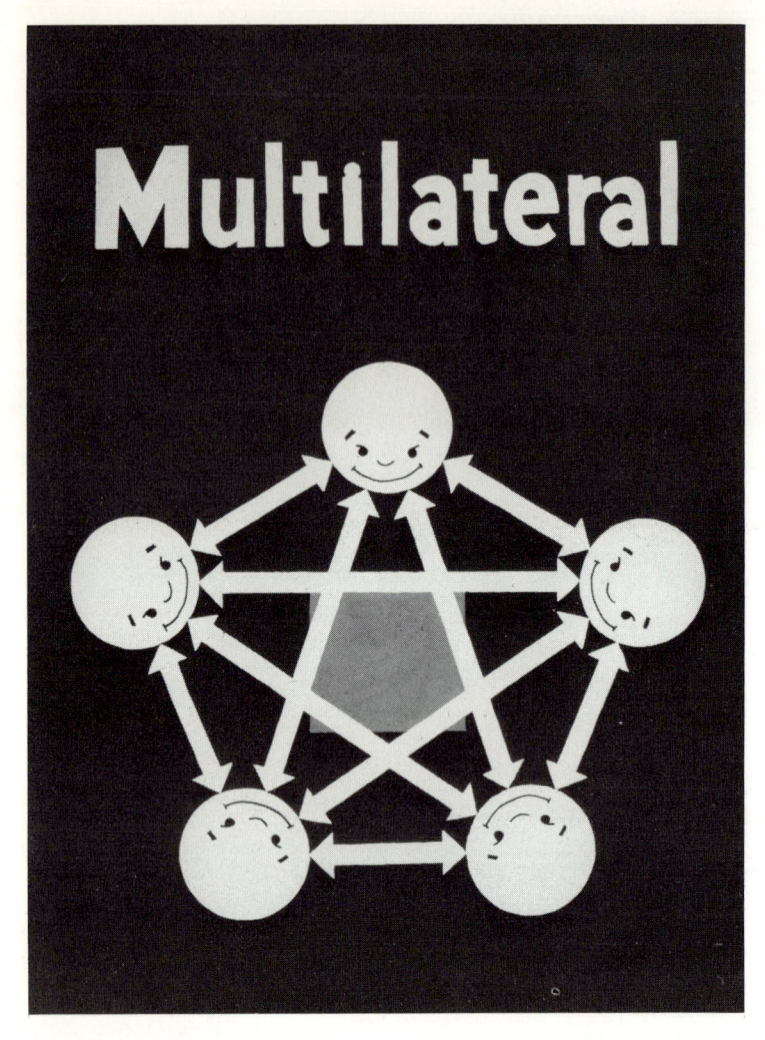

PROCESS VI. MULTILATERAL

Action of a competitive nature among three or more persons, with no one person as an antagonist. This process is typical of a poker game, and often is the major modus operandi of many adults. (See Figure 6.)

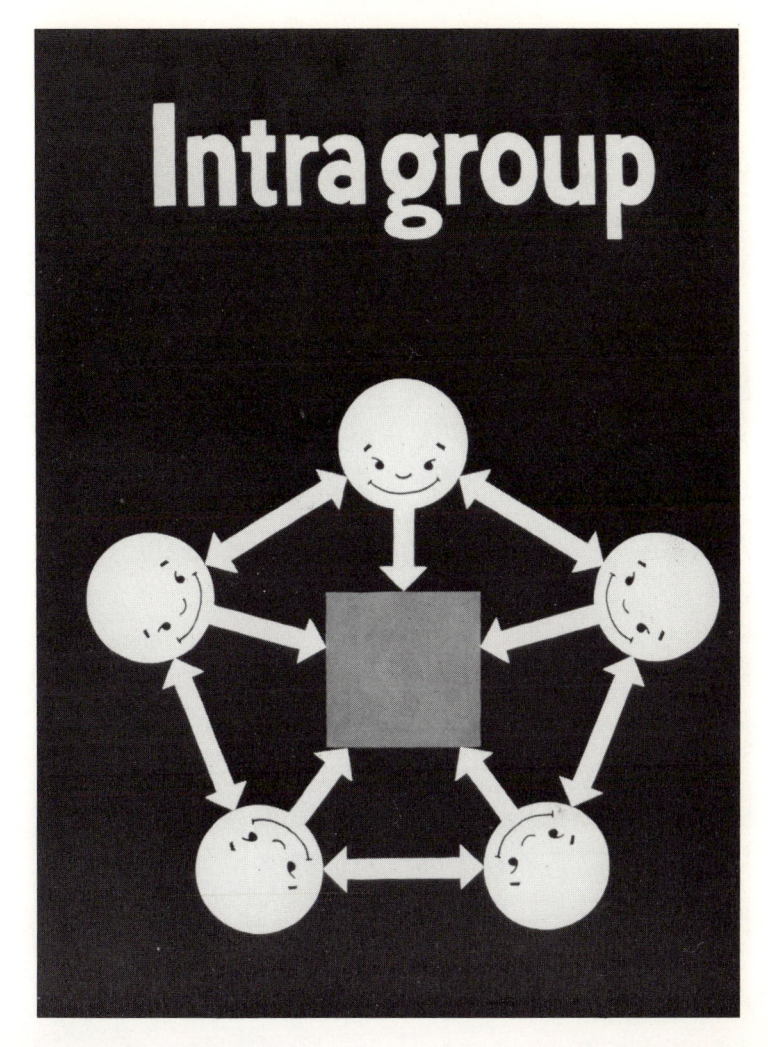

PROCESS VII. INTRAGROUP

Action of a *cooperative* nature by two or more persons intent upon reaching a mutual goal. Action requires positive verbal and nonverbal interaction. This is the process required in interview structures and in a variety of activities such as playing in a band, singing in a choir, acting in a play. This is a true group structure. It requires the interactive process known as *cohesion;* i.e., when people in the group can resolve conflict through compromise, thus enabling the group to develop and express positive feelings for one another. The opposite process is *anomie;* i.e., when people in the group cannot resolve conflict and cannot continue the activity; anomie is the inability of the participants to "give and take" and to get along with one another by arriving at a compromise. (See Figure 7.)

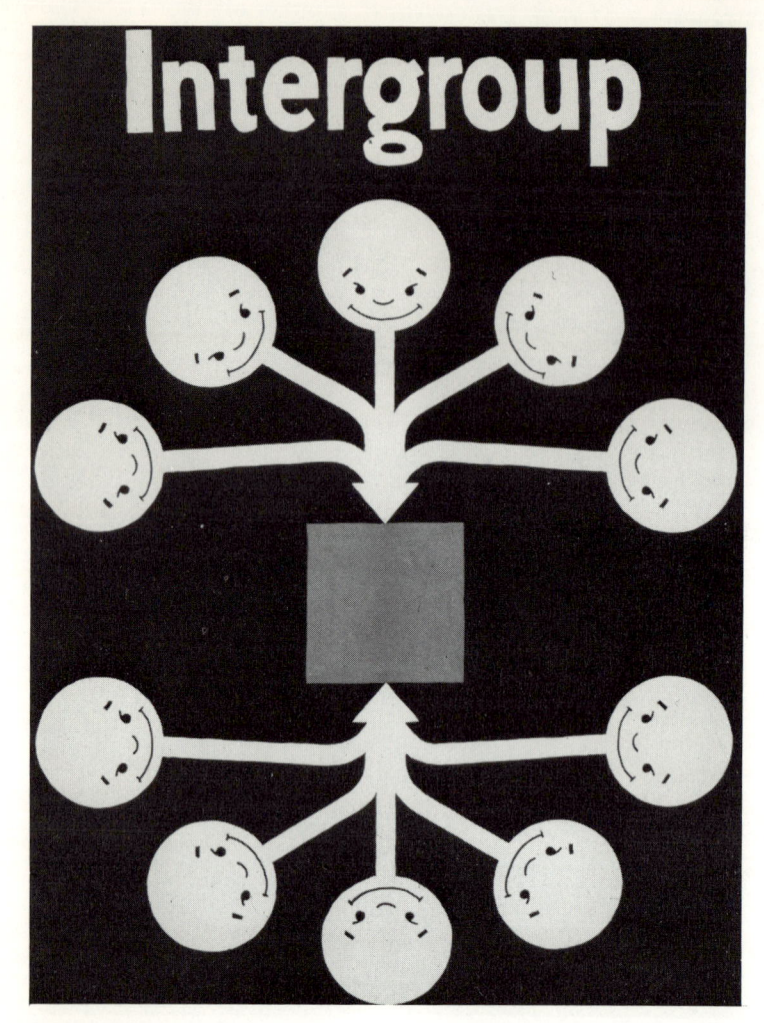

170   *Social and Behavioral Factors in Programming*

PROCESS VIII. INTERGROUP

    Action of a competitive nature between two ore more intragroups. This process is inherent in team games such as basketball or bridge. Unfortunately, participants who have been unable to relate or who lack experience in an *intragroup* structure are prematurely involved in *inter*group activity. Often what they need is a positive *aggregate* experience rather than a premature attempt in a true group experience. When a participant has not been meeting with considerable success in an intragroup structure over a period of time, he cannot be expected to meet with success as a member of a team in the intergroup structure. (See Figure 8.)

When participants are involved in the *intragroup* processes prematurely, they manifest certain negative behaviors. Some of these are:

Counterdependency—When someone in the group wants everyone to think that he does not rely on anyone else's judgment in order to make a decision, and he goes overboard to prove this, he is said to be counterdependent. ("The lady doth protest too much, methinks" Hamlet, act 3, sc. 2, line 242.) In reality, this person has not accepted his need to rely on others. The mature adult recognizes he has some degree of need to be dependent upon others.

Dependency—When someone in the group is continually influenced by others in the group and takes little or no independent action, he is said to be dependent. Sometimes this behavior is manifested by two or three individuals who will always caucus before making a decision or won't become involved in an activity without the others. When two people do this it is called "pairing"; three or more are referred to as a "clique." Although maturity includes some degree of dependence, true maturity means interdependence; that is, the ability to recognize and respond as well to the needs of others to be dependent upon us.

Fight—When someone in the group becomes anxious or upset and he challenges persons in the group who are upsetting him. The more they try to persuade him, the more he resists and the more violently he "fights." This usually is on a verbal level, but could degenerate to a physical level.

Flight—When someone in the group becomes anxious or upset and withdraws from conflict with persons in the group who are upsetting him. The more they try to urge him toward a decision or action, the more he withdraws. This is on a verbal level, but could degenerate to a physical level and the person could walk out of the group session.

In mature group interaction, there is opposition and accommodation between participants in a group. When opposition occurs, accommodation is sought through the following processes:

Elimination—Argument and combat, each faction seeking to win, and finally one faction or individual withdrawing.

Subjugation—Argument and combat resulting in a dominant faction that forces the others to accept its point of view.

Compromise—Argument and combat between approximately equal subgroups, cliques, or individuals, resulting in each giving up something to safeguard the activity.

Alliance—Argument and expression of independence, but combining of forces to achieve a common goal.

Integration—Argument and discussion with all of the participants arriving at a solution that is better than any single solution. This is true "cohesion."

Thus in therapeutic recreation service, knowledge of the dynamics of group life becomes an important factor in order to program effectively with respect to clinical goals. It becomes obvious that an inappropriate program structure and interactive process can not only be counterindicated in working with patients and clients who have special needs, but could result in fostering regressive behavior and undermining the work of the rest of the clinical staff.[1]

---

[1] Some general readings in group dynamics include M. and H. Knowles, *Introduction to Group Dynamics* (New York: Association Press, 1959); M. B. Miles, *Learning to Work in Groups* (New York: Teachers College Press, 1959). More advanced readings include A. P. Hare, E. F. Borgatta, and R. F. Bales, *Small Groups* (New York: Alfred A. Knopf, 1966); D. Stock and H. A. Thelen, *Emotional Dynamics and Group Culture* (Washington, D.C.: National Education Association, 1958); J. W. Thibaut and H. H. Kelley, *The Social Psychology of Groups* (New York: John Wiley and Sons, 1959); and D. Cartwright and A. Zander, *Group Dynamics* (New York: Harper and Row, 1960).

11
Social and Behavioral Factors in Program Content

There are numerous sources one may turn to for typical material concerning program content. Content can include popular recreative activities or more esoteric and personal activities. The specialist can choose from the infinite number of activities people engage in when they play leisure roles. There are a number of sources in the literature which indicate that certain activities appear more successful when programming for patients or clients who have specific limitations. A bibliography that includes examples of some of these sources appears at the end of this chapter.

With respect to a goal orientation, therapeutic recreation specialists must understand more about an activity than is contained in the usual "how to do it" information. The following material discusses some of the social and behavioral aspects of program content which are important in therapeutic recreation service.

A popular activity used for recreative purposes may be viewed as a singular artifact of civilization in that it is replicable. You and I might participate in the activity today, and tomorrow others might participate in the very same activity. The activity can be viewed as a discrete entity or a system that incorporates a matrix of identifiable inherent elements—elements that may be manipulated with respect to clinical goals. Some of these elements relate to the physical structure and processes associated with the activity per se, and they do not alter unless participants decide to alter them, while other elements relate to the participant's behavior. The purist will declare that once an element in the matrix is altered, we are no longer dealing with the same entity. Thus an activity such as basketball played in wheelchairs is not basketball but another activity, and should have a different name. It is true that most participants make slight alterations in activity elements to suit their immediate participation needs, and usually these alterations are minimal. It has been suggested that when a recreation specialist makes a major alteration in an activity, it is demeaning to participants to suggest that they are engaging in the original activity because the same name is being used. The following material delineates the elements of the matrix and discusses the potential for manipulation and alteration.

Activity Elements

All activity has a *purpose,* an intent, an aim. In weaving, it is to make a piece of cloth; in poker, it is to draw the best hand; in swimming, it is to successfully move through the water. In order to effectively participate in a specified activity, one must understand its purpose or the goal one aspires to. Patients or clients who have a disordered sensorium because of illness or medication, or who have experienced a physical trauma such as a cerebral vascular accident, or who have a degree of mental retardation, or who lack knowledge of the activity because of social deprivation may experience difficulty in participation because they do not have a clear conception of the purpose of the activity. It then becomes the responsibility of the therapeutic recreation specialist to either insure that they understand the purpose of the activity or that the purpose be altered so that they can conceptualize the intent of action.

For every activity there is a specified *procedure for action,* or a "how to do it." In some activities, such as shuffleboard, the procedure is not very complicated, while in other activities, such as knitting, it may be quite complex. The procedure for action is a series of specified operations and required courses of action that move the participant toward the goal or purpose of the activity. The specialist can alter procedures as necessary. When the procedure is complicated and requires considerable concentration and potential participants have limited attention spans, alteration in procedure may be necessary. However alteration may also be necessary when the procedure is too repetitive and participants may become easily bored or distracted. Physical limitations sometimes require alteration of procedures, and at times require maximum alteration which changes the entire nature of the activity.

Each activity includes *rules governing action.* These fixed principles determine conduct and standards of behavior in an activity. They confine or limit the procedures for action. Rules may be minimal or elaborate. For example, there are a few rules one must remember when playing bridge. These rules are known as bridge "etiquette"—violations engender score penalties. However, in a craft shop there are no standard sets of rules, and often for safety's sake a specialist must develop an elaborate set of explicit rules. In contrast, participants at a movie or a play or other popular social functions are expected to "know the rules." Often this is not the case. Because of illness they may have known the rules and have now forgotten them. Certain activities may be new experiences for some who never have had an opportunity to learn the rules. In some situations, psychic factors militate against "playing by the rules." It is the responsibility of the specialist to insure that participants know and understand rules governing action, or else he should modify rules as the situation requires.

In addition to the purpose, procedures, and rules, some activities require a fixed *number of participants* while other activities do not. In team games, the number of participants is specified, and usually the minimum number and the maximum number are identical. At a community sing, any number present can sing, and those who don't wish to sing do not have to participate. In this latter situation, nonparticipation does not affect the course of the action for participants. However, when a fourth for bridge cannot be found, action cannot proceed. It is necessary for the specialist to select activities that will accommodate the participants who want to engage in activity, and not be in a position of stimulating interest and finding that there are not enough participants for a chosen activity. This has the effect of weakening a relationship with those patients or clients who were stimulated. The converse may also be true; that is, if an activity is chosen that could involve an unlimited number of participants, care must be exercised to avoid overstimulation. In that event, too many participants in a single activity at the same time may decrease the amount of satisfaction derived from the activity. This can clearly be seen when a swimming pool is too crowded, or a dance has too many people on the dance floor at the same time.

Another element present in activity is the *role of participants*. In some activities the role or indicated functions and status are the same, while in others, the role and subsequent power function may be different. For example, at a social dance, all participants have the same roles (one follows and one leads), but in a theatrical presentation, usually only one person has the "lead." In a craft shop, someone may be designated as the "tool librarian" (a unique status), while in the game of chess both players have the same status. This element of activity lends itself to manipulation for clinical purposes. The specialist is in a position of assigning roles in order to enhance the status of a patient or client, or to generate certain positive or negative feelings that can be made explicit.

Similarly, another activity element, *results or payoff,* can serve the same manipulative functions. Results are the values assigned to the outcome of action, or the fulfilling of the purpose. The specialist can place great value upon the person who has produced something, or who has won, or who has accomplished a difficult task. The specialist can also play down the results in the interest of a clinical goal, highlighting other behavioral aspects as being more important. A result can be a prize, a medal, mention in an in-house journal, money, an extra dessert, or any item or response of value in a specific setting.

Two additional elements that may or may not be specified in all activities are the *physical setting and environmental requirements,* and *required equipment.* These elements are a function of the logistics of the program and the limitations or lack of limitations that a patient or client brings to the activity. Both factors may be altered or manipulated to enhance or limit participation.

The final element in the activity matrix that must be considered is the specified *abilities and skills required for participation.* Each activity requires different human abilities and skills for participation in a recreative activity. The following material presents a brief discussion of aspects of the three behavioral domains and their relationship to recreative involvement, which one must understand before considering this final element in the matrix.

Although participation in any activity requires the utilization of skills and abilities in each of the three behavioral domains, it is theoretically possible to examine each of the three domains separately. In fact, many people consider that physical impairment only affects the *sensory-motor* domain, mental retardation and related neurological impairments affect the *cognitive* domain, and mental illness affects the *affective* domain. This of course is not true, inasmuch as there are signs and symptoms of disturbance in all aspects of personality when one of the domains is impaired. However, it is important to understand the theories and concepts regarding behavioral domains, because it is true that the primary disorder is usually in one domain. When a disorder results in a permanent impairment and consequently a permanent disability, it is necessary to understand how to avoid asking a patient or client to use skills and abilities that are impaired. To do this, the recreation specialist must understand which skills and abilities are required for participation in any given activity. He must have a system for classifying activities that will help him to do this.

Sensory-Motor Domain

There is much in the behavioral literature about the domains. Considerable work has been done in studying the *sensory-motor* domain. Much of the literature of physical and occupational therapy deals with this type of information. The sensory-motor domain includes such factors as bodily movement, manipulative motor skills, coordination, sequences and patterning of movements, endurance, sight, hearing, balance, strength, and other related aspects. It must be recognized that some sensory ability is required for all activity participation; however, it is possible for persons with severe sensory limitations, such as both deafness and blindness, to engage in a variety of recreation activities.[1]

To determine which aspects of the sensory-motor domain are involved in a specific recreation activity, a kinesiological analysis would be conducted. After,

---

[1] See Irving Miller, *Recreation Services for Deaf-Blind Persons* (New York: Industrial Home for the Blind, 1959); and Donna Verstrate, *Social Group Work with Deaf-Blind Adults* (New York: American Foundation for the Blind, 1959).

this analysis is applied to the condition of a specific patient or client. No two persons with impairment have the same limitations. Fortunately, many popular recreative activities have been subjected to kinesiological analysis, and some activities have been tested electromyographically. These analyses appear in the literature.[2]

A complete sensory-motor analysis of an activity would include data concerning each of the body's physical systems:

bronchopulmonary
cardiovascular
digestive
endocrine
hemic and lymphatic
integumentary
metabolic
musculoskeletal
nervous
reproductive
sensory
urogenital

However, most kinesiological analyses primarily concern musculoskeletal activity per se, and concentrate on positions and movements of parts of the body, essential physical skills, joint and muscle involvement, and often discuss environmental aids or interferences with movement. Fundamental movements of the body have been studied for a long time, and as a consequence, a standard classification system has been in use to describe these movements. The taxonomy is offered here as a matter of information:

abduction	moving away from the midline of the body
adduction	moving toward the midline of the body
alignment	segments in a straight line
circumduction	moving in a circular path or moving in a cone shape
depression	lowering of the shoulder
elevation	raising of the shoulder
extension	straight alignment
external rotation	circular movement away from the body
flexion	segments approach each other by bending or retracting
hyperextension	beyond alignment, or beyond the starting point

[2]For example, see M. G. Scott, *Analysis of Human Motion* (New York: Appleton-Century-Crofts, 1963).

internal rotation	circular movement toward the body
lateral flexion	bending of the head or trunk
locomotion	movement of the entire body from one place to another
opposition	position of the thumb opposite the fingers
pronation	to turn face down
protraction	another word for extension
retraction	another word for flexion
rotation	circular movement of the head
supernation	to turn face up

Joint movement is measured in degrees of the circle. Thus when the shoulder joint is at a 90-degree angle, the arm is parallel to the floor and is extended in a straight line from the shoulder. If the arm is raised in a straight line over the head, the shoulder angle would be 180 degrees. The following is a partial example of a kinesiological analysis of the sport of archery.

Archery

(Descriptions of the positions and movements refer to right-handed persons. For left-handed persons, positioning and movement of head and neck, trunk, and lower extremities is, in most instances, the reverse of those presented here.)

I. Parts of the Body: Positions and Movements Required
   A. Head and Neck
      1. *Position*—Head rotated at right angle to shoulder, eyes focused on target.
      2. *Movement*—Immobile while drawing bowstring and releasing the arrow.
      3. *Purpose*—Enables archer to take aim.
      4. *External Conditions*—No obstruction to line of vision between archer and target.
   B. Trunk
      1. *Position*—Trunk erect, rotated at lateral angle to target.
      2. *Movement*—Immobile while drawing bowstring and releasing arrow.
      3. *Purpose*—Permits proper positioning of arms.
      4. *External Conditions*—Clothing of proper design and size to avoid interference in assuming and maintaining required position.
   C. Upper Extremities
      1. *Position*—(a) Bow arm: forefinger and thumb of left hand hold bow at "the grip," bow rests against palm and fleshy base of thumb. Left arm extended almost straight (but not locked in extension) holding bow perpendicular to ground. Left hand is nearly at shoulder height. (b) Arrow arm: forefinger and thumb of right hand hold feathered end of arrow perpendicular to bowstring. Right arm extended and flexed across upper chest; with right hand near left shoulder; just

below chin. Point of arrow rests on the "V" formed by thumb and forefinger of hand holding the bow.
  2. *Movement*—(a) The "draw": forefinger, second finger, and third finger of right hand hold bowstring. Right forefinger and second finger hold arrow against bowstring. Left arm and hand extended with wrist pronated as bow is held up and out toward target. As fingers of right hand draw bowstring back, left wrist is supernated. Bowstring touches center of chin; fingers, hand, wrist, and elbow of right arm are in a straight line with the arrow. Right and left scapulae upwardly rotated and adducted during draw. (b) The "release": bowstring slips from fingers of right hand, right arm moves back at shoulder level. Left wrist resumes former pronated position. Both scapulae remain in adduction.
  3. *Purpose*—Impart momentum and control direction of arrow's movement toward target.
  4. *External Conditions*—Size and weight of bow, tension of bowstring, distance from target determine: (a) amount of energy expended during contraction and relaxation of hand and arm muscles; (b) widening and narrowing of intraarticular spaces between various joints of the upper extremities.
 D. Lower Extremities
  1. *Position*—Feet apart (about 7 to 12 inches) to balance the body directly over the shooting line. Weight distributed equally, knees slightly flexed.
  2. *Movement*—Immobile while drawing bowstring and releasing arrow.
  3. *Purpose*—Support and balance trunk.
  4. *External Conditions*—A flat, dry, smooth but not slippery surface to stand on makes it easier for archer to assume and maintain the necessary stance.
II. Esential Physical Skills
 A. *Sensory*
 Sufficient: (a) vision to sight a target; (b) tactile sense to feel relative positions of bow, arrow; and (c) kinesthetic sense to perceive muscular motion, distribution of body weight, state of equilibrium.
 B. *Respiratory*
 The ability to control breathing affects balance, maintenance of bodily position, and the sequence of movements involved in aiming, holding the bow and arrow steady, drawing bowstring, releasing arrow.
 C. *Musculoskeletal*
 Ability to: (a) produce fairly strong action of flexors and extensors on the right side of the trunk, with corresponding control of those on left; (b) rotate head in the necessary direction and hold it steady; (c) coordinate action of the musculature of upper back and shoulder girdle; (d) keep arms in position, and control digital manipulation of bow, bowstring, and arrow. The ability to stand up is not essential. With minor adaptations, it is possible to perform successfully from a sitting position.

III. Joints and Muscles Involved
   A. Head and Neck
   The head held erect and rotated to the left (right-handed archer); muscles involved include:

   Splenius cervicis and capitis (left)
   Sacrospinalis cervicis and capitis (left)
   Occipitofrontalis (left)
   Occipitoventor (right)
   Multifidus cervicus portion (right)
   Sternocleidomastoideus (right)
   Subclavius
   Obliquus abdominis externus
   Obliquus abdominis internus
   Rectus abdominis
   Quadratus lumborum
   Psoas major and minor
   Rotatores spinae
   Interspinales
   Intertransversarii
   Levatores costarum
   Spinalis dorsi

   B. Trunk
   The same muscles and joints erect in a standing (or sitting) position are used to maintain the rigidity of the trunk which is necessary for archery. In the standing position, the hips are abducted and extended. The following muscles are used:

   Gluteus medius (posterior fibers)
   Gluteus minimus (posterior fibers)
   Tensor fasciae latae
   Gluteus maximus (upper fibers)

   The scapula is upwardly rotated and adducted during the draw, with continued adduction during the release of arrow. The following muscles are used:

   Trapezius
   Rhomboideus (major and minor)
   Serratus anterior
   Subclavius
   Pectoralis minor

   C. Upper Extremities

   (a) The bow arm: humerus slightly abducted and inwardly rotated; forearm flexed and pronated; wrist in ulnar flexion; thumb flexed and in opposition to the index finger; fingers flexed and adducted. Muscles involved include:

   Deltoids
   Supraspinatus

Infraspinatus biceps
Trapezius
Subclavius
Teres minor
Teres major
Triceps
Extensor carpi radialis (longus and brevis)
Flexor carpi (radialis and ulnaris)

(b) The arrow arm: humerus in dorsal abduction; forearm flexed and pronated; thumb flexed and in opposition to the index finger, index finger flexed. Muscles involved include:

Subscapularis
Teres major
Latissimus dorsi
Coracobrachialis
Serratus
Pectoralis minor
Deltoid
Pectoralis major
Flexors (elbow)
Pronator teres biceps

Positions during the draw include:

(a) The bow arm: scapula upwardly rotated and adducted; humerus horizontally extended and inwardly rotated; forearm slightly flexed and pronated; wrist in radial flexion; thumb flexed and opposing the index finger; index and other fingers flexed and adducted.

(b) The arrow arm: scapula upwardly rotated and beginning to adduct; humerus horizontally flexed, elevated, and inwardly rotated; forearm flexed and pronated; wrist in extension; thumb flexed and hyperadducted.

Positions during the release include:

Left scapula in continued adduction; left humerus in horizontal extension and inward rotation; forearm slightly flexed and pronated, wrist in ulnar flexion; fingers and thumb flexed and adducted. Right scapula in continued adduction; right humerus in continued horizontal extension.

D. Lower Extremities

The feet are placed in anatomic position; with knees slightly flexed. Major muscles involved are:

Biceps femoris
Semitendinosus
Semimembranosus
Sartorius
Popliteus
Gastrocnemius

IV. Aids or Interferences

A light bow (under 18 lbs.) requires less power and strength for the draw. Special gloves, arm guards, and finger tabs are useful to protect skin surfaces. The shorter bows and arrows available for archers of small stature are helpful to people with limited muscular strength and those unable to stand.

Although recreation specialists do not normally have this amount of detail available concerning most program activities, it can be seen that using this material in conjunction with information regarding a patient or client's impairment enables the specialist to eliminate those program activites which require use of an impaired physical ability, thus insuring greater participation for the patient or client population.

To enable the reader to further understand the complexity of bodily movement with respect to recreative activity, the following material by Wickwire is included.[3] Personnel in physical and occupational therapy would use this information to respond to a physician's prescription for treatment of pathology. They would have this information at their fingertips, and would be experienced in using it. Personnel in therapeutic recreation service would not use this information for treatment of a pathological condition, but rather as a way of understanding how to *avoid* involving a patient or client in an activity that requires use of a muscle or joint that is impaired. The specialist would attempt to involve a patient or client in an activity in which he would not be limited, but would meet with success.

Activity Analysis For Rehabilitation
George C. Wickwire

The purpose of this analysis of activities is to suggest various crafts and games which may be used to assist in rehabilitation of the disabled. Activities should be chosen with care to increase the motion of joints, to improve muscular strength, or to develop specific coordinations, according to the needs of each individual case. A possible advantage of exercising a muscle in several different activities is that some motor units of a muscle may be used when it contracts in one combination and other motor units used when it contracts in another combination.

1. Thumb: Flexion

    Muscles involved—Flexor pollicis longus; Flexor pollicis brevis; Adductor pollicis, and Oppenens Pollicis.

[3] Reprinted with permission of the American Congress of Physical Medicine and Rehabilitation, from *The Archives of Physical Medicine and Rehabilitation* (September 1955), pp. 578-86.

Social and Behavioral Factors in Program Content

ACTIVITY USED	MOTION INDICATED
pottery	pinching clay
topography	grasping type
hammering	grasping handle
sawing	grasping handle
gardening	flexing thumb to pull weeds and hold tools
typing	striking space bar
piano playing	striking keys
card weaving	turning cards, combing, and tying knots
tennis	grasping racket
reading	turning pages
leather	lacing
writing	holding pencil
jacks	grasping jacks
stringed instrument	plucking strings
knitting	holding needles
darts	grasping darts
ring toss	grasping rings

2. Thumb: Extension

   Muscles involved—Extensor pollicis longus and Extensor pollicis brevis.

darts	release dart
marbles	picking up marbles
ring toss	flinging hand open
typing	release space bar
cutting	opening scissors
knitting	release needle
loom weaving	combing warp, placing shuttle through
woodworking	sanding with a block
basket weave	grasping materials
cards	dealing

3. Thumb: Abduction

   Muscles involved—Abductor pollicis longus; Abductor pollicis brevis; Opponens pollicis, and Extensor pollicis brevis.

embroidery	spreading and untangling
weaving	combing warp
leather	releasing tools
jewelry	releasing tools
shuffleboard	picking up puck
checkers	grasping and releasing checkers

4. Thumb: Adduction

   Muscles involved—Adductor pollicis and Flexor pollicis longus.

pottery	pinching pots
leather	grasping tools
gardening	grasping tools
cards	dealing and drawing cards
woodworking	holding tools
card weaving	shifting cards
sewing	grasping needle
jewelry	grasping tools

5. Thumb: Opposition

   Muscle involved—Opponens pollicis.

weaving	separating reeds
writing	holding pencil
gardening	holding tools
reading	turning pages
cat's cradle	holding string
pottery	throwing at the wheel
crocheting	holding needles
shuffleboard	holding puck
ring toss	holding rings
ping pong	holding paddle
hockey	holding stick

6. Fingers (2nd, 3rd, 4th, 5th): Flexion

   Muscles involved—Flexor digitorum profundus; Flexor digitorum sublimus; Flexor digit; Quinti brevis; Opponens digiti quinti; Abductor digiti quinti; Lumbricales; Interossi dorsales, and Interossi volares.

sewing	grasping needles and threads
weaving	pulling treadles, shuttle, warping, beating, combing, threading
woodworking	grasping tools
pottery	pinching and squeezing clay
drawing	grasping brushes and pencils
carving	grasping and holding object and tools
darts	grasping darts
gardening	grasping rake, hoe, etc.
musical instrument	moving fingers over air outlets, or plucking, strumming, etc.
typing	pressing keys

7. Fingers (2nd 3rd, 4th): Extension

   Muscles involved—Extensor digitorum communis; Extensor indicis proprius; Lumbricales; Interossi dorsales, and Interossi volares.

needlework	grasping, cutting, etc.
weaving	beating, combing

Social and Behavioral Factors in Program Content

woodwork	manipulating tools
carving	sanding
drawing	manipulating implements
bowling	releasing ball
darts	releasing darts
ring toss	releasing ring
typing	releasing pressure on keys

8. Fingers (2nd, 3rd, 4th): Adduction

   Muscles involved—Flexor digitorum profundus and Interossi volares.

weaving	combing warp
woodworking	sanding and polishing
pottery	pinching and molding
ball games	grasping ball

9. Fingers (2nd, 3rd, 4th): Abduction

   Muscles involved—Interossi dorsales; Abductor digiti quinti; Lumbricales, and Extensor digitorum communis.

needlework	spreading and untangling thread
ringtoss	releasing ring
checkers	releasing checkers
piano playing	reaching for keys
ball games	catching and holding ball

10. Wrist: Flexion

    Muscles involved—Flexor carpi radialis; Flexor carpi ulnaris, and Palmaris longus.

woodwork	hammering, polishing, painting
pottery	wedging, throwing at wheel
ball games	throwing
darts	throwing
badminton	swinging racket
tennis	swinging racket
carving	grasping tools
writing	moving implements

11. Wrist: Extension

    Muscles involved—Extensor carpi radialis longus; Extensor carpi radialis brevis, and Extensor carpi ulnaris.

dice	releasing dice
tennis	returning high serve

186   *Social and Behavioral Factors in Programming*

        ball games   catching ball
        pottery   rolling clay
        woodwork   sanding, holding down objects, hammering

12. **Wrist: Radial Deviation**

    Muscles involved—Flexor carpi radialis and Extensor carpi radialis longus.

        carving   grasping tools
        string instrument   strumming, plucking
        fly casting   throwing rod line out
        woodwork   polishing
        horseshoes   releasing object

13. **Wrist: Ulnar Deviation**

    Muscles involved—Flexor carpi ulnaris and Extensor carpi ulnaris.

        musical instrument   strumming, releasing fingers over outlets
        fly casting   throwing line over back and casting
        woodwork   polishing

14. **Forearm: Supination**

    Muscles involved—Biceps brachii and Supinator.

        weaving   threading the loom
        jewelry   polishing on wheel
        leather   lacing
        ping pong   hitting ball
        fishing   casting
        cards   dealing and drawing
        reading   turning pages
        pottery   wedging

15. **Forearm: Pronation**

    Muscles involved—Pronator teres and Pronator quadratus.

        woodwork   driving screws, chiseling
        basketball   dribbling, shooting
        weaving   warping, threading, beating weft
        music   string instruments
        jewelry   soldering
        bookbinding   glueing
        square-dancing   twirls

Social and Behavioral Factors in Program Content

16. Forearm: Flexion

    Muscles involved—Brachialis; Biceps brachii; Brachioradialis, and Pronator teres.

archery	drawing the string
baseball	pitching, batting, catching
golf	driving and putting
rowing	pulling back on the oars
swimming	breaststroke, sidestroke
tennis	serving and smashing
weaving	beating, winding, threading
woodwork	sawing, hammering, sanding
jewelry	polishing
cards	dealing and drawing
pottery	wedging, rolling
gardening	lifting, pulling

17. Forearm: Extension

    Muscles involved—Triceps brachii and Anconeus.

bowling	at start of approach
tennis	serving and playing
volleyball	hitting the ball
horseshoes	throwing the shoe
ping pong	hitting the ball
basketball	dribbling, passing, shooting
cards	putting cards on table
weaving	threading the loom, winding yarn
woodwork	hammering, sawing
softball	throwing, batting
swimming	sidestroke, front crawl, breaststroke
gardening	raking, hoeing
boxing	punching
canoeing	paddling
fencing	thrusting
fishing	casting

18. Arm: Flexion

    Muscles involved—Deltoid (anterior); Coracobrachialis; Biceps brachii, and Pectoralis major (clavicular).

Basketry	pulling out reed from skeins
horseshoes	releasing shoes
leatherwork	lacing, tooling
pottery	wedging

woodwork	sawing, planing, sanding, hammering
ping pong	swinging paddle
ring toss	throwing rings
shuffleboard	thrust forward, and passively relaxing
rowing	pulling on oars
swimming	front crawl, most strokes
softball	pitching

19. Arm: Extension

    Muscles involved—Deltoid (posterior); Latissimus dorsi, and Teres major.

woodwork	sawing, sanding, filing, planing
horseshoes	throwing shoes
ring toss	pulling arm back to throw
swimming	backstroke
rowing	pulling on oars
ping pong	hitting ball
skipping rope	turning rope
baseball	pitching, batting
shot put	before release
tennis	swinging racket
golf	putting

20. Arm: Medial Rotation

    Muscles involved—Teres major; Subscapularis; Pectoralis major; Latissimus dorsi, and Coracobrachialis.

weaving	putting shuttle through shed
pottery	pouring, wedging
woodwork	driving screws
tennis	swing racket
baseball	pitching, throwing
ring toss	releasing ring
swimming	strokes
skipping rope	turning

21. Arm: Lateral Rotation

    Muscles involved—Teres minor; Infraspinatus, and Deltoid (posterior).

woodwork	driving screws
horseshoes	throwing shoes
leatherwork	lacing
ping pong	swinging paddle
baseball	batting, pitching
fencing	thrusting
tennis	hitting ball
swimming	crawl

Social and Behavioral Factors in Program Content   189

22. Arm: Abduction

    Muscles involved—Supraspinatus and Deltoid (middle).

shuffleboard	picking up pucks
archery	drawing bow
swimming	breaststroke
tennis	serving and front stroke
volleyball	hitting ball when above shoulder
baseball	side arm pitching
cards	dealing
badminton	hitting bird
fishing	casting

23. Arm: Adduction

    Muscles involved—Pectoralis major; Teres major; Teres minor; Infraspinatus; Coracobrachialis; Triceps (long head), and Latissimus dorsi.

shuffleboard	picking up pucks
pottery	throwing on wheel
woodwork	sawing, planing
golf	swinging and carry through
baseball	batting
tennis	backstroke
canoeing	propelling phase
billiards	stroking cue

24. Shoulder Girdle: Upward Rotation

    Muscles involved—Trapezius (1 and 2) and Serratus anterior.

woodwork	sawing, hammering
weaving	winding warp on board
ceramics	wedging
volleyball	hitting ball above head
tennis	serving and smashing
basketball	shooting, reaching, jumping
rowing	pulling oars toward you
baseball	batting, pitching

25. Shoulder Girdle: Downward Rotation

    Muscles involved—Rhomboids; Levator scapula, and Pectoralis minor.

woodwork	hammering, sawing
swimming	crawl
weaving	winding warp on board
ceramics	wedging

tennis	downward force on ball in serve
rowing	pushing oars away
bowling	releasing ball
baseball	batting and pitching

26. Shoulder Girdle: Abduction

    Muscles involved—Pectoralis minor and Serratus anterior.

swimming	crawl, breaststroke
tennis	follow through on stroke
baseball	pitching, throwing, batting
gardening	raking, hoeing, mowing
woodwork	sanding, planing
fencing	thrust, lunge

27. Shoulder Girdle: Adduction

    Muscles involved—Trapezius (3 and 4), Rhomboids.

weaving	beating
gardening	raking, hoeing
art	large-scale drawing
swimming	backstroke, breaststroke, crawl
tennis	swinging arms backward
archery	drawing bow
baseball	swinging bat, throwing ball

28. Shoulder Girdle: depression

    Muscles involved—Pectoralis minor; Subclavius, and Trapezius.

woodwork	sawing
ceramics	wheel throwing
weaving	winding warp
tennis	forceful follow through
bowling	approach to ball release
shuffleboard	forward thrust

29. Shoulder Girdle: Elevation

    Muscles involved—Trapezius (1 and 2); Levator scapula and Rhomboids.

woodwork	sawing, carrying lumber
bowling	lifting ball
weaving	carding wool, beating
tennis	smashing, serving
volleyball	reaching to hit ball

swimming	crawl
basketball	jumping and shooting

30. Head and Neck: Extension

    Muscles involved—Splenius capitis and Semispinalis capitis.

ring toss	tossing rings
basketball	shooting and throwing
badminton	swinging at bird
skeet shooting	follow high bird
discus	releasing discus
softball	pitching, throwing
archery	drawing bow
horseshoes	releasing shoes
tennis	swinging
golf	following through
swimming	holding head above water
painting	up and down strokes

31. Head and Neck: Flexion

    Muscles involved—Sternocleidomastoideus; Platysma; Rectus capitis anterior; Rectus capitis lateralis; Longus capitis; Longus colli; Scalenus anterior; Scalenus medius, and Scalenus posterior.

tennis	swinging through
golf	putting and driving
woodwork	sawing, hammering
shotput	throwing shot
violin	holding under chin
swimming	overhead stroke
billiards	looking down when stroking
ping pong	swinging paddle
ring toss	picking up rings
shuffleboard	thrusting forward

32. Head and Neck: Rotation

    Muscles involved—Sternocleidomastoideus; Splenius capitis; Semispinalis capitis; Rectus capitis anterior; Rectus capitis lateralis; Longus capitis; Longus colli, and Trapezius (clavicular).

tennis	watching game
baseball	batting
weaving	watching pattern and pedals
archery	sighting aim
high jump	clearing bar

33. Head and Neck: Lateral Flexion

    Muscles involved—Sternocleidomastoideus; Scalenus anterior; Scalenus medius; Scalenus posterior; Rectus capitus lateralis.

violin	holding violin
baseball	batting
archery	aiming
swimming	moving head side to side
pole vault	running with pole
discus	approach
fishing	casting
golf	follow through

34. Spinal Column: Flexion

    Muscles involved—Rectus abdominis; External oblique; Internal oblique; Psoas major, and Iliacus.

bowling	rolling ball
ball games	throwing, catching, hitting
cycling	bending forward
dancing	leaning forward
horseshoes	throwing shoes
swimming	kicking, flexing, floating
gardening	shoveling, spading, raking
rowboating	rowing
shuffleboard	pushing disk

35. Spinal Column: Extension

    Muscles involved—Sacrospinalis; Multifidus, and Quadratus lumborum.

billiards	rackshot
ball games	catching, throwing, hitting
football	kicking
horseshoes	throwing shoes
darts	throwing
tennis	hitting with racket
dancing	bending backwards, dip
swimming	backstroke, floating
fencing	thrusting

36. Spinal Column: Lateral Flexion

    Muscles involved—Quadratus lumborum; Levatores costarum; Sacrospinalis; Iliacus; Psoas major; Latissimus dorsi; Internal oblique; External oblique, and Rectus abdominis.

Social and Behavioral Factors in Program Content

billiards	shooting at ball
bowling	rolling ball
ball games	passing, throwing, hitting
golf	hitting ball
gardening	planting, weeding, raking
canoeing	paddling
shuffleboard	pushing disk
swimming	sidestroke
darts	throwing
horseshoes	tossing shoes
jacks	grabbing jacks
dancing	swaying, rotating

37. Spinal Column: Rotation

    Muscles involved—External oblique; Levatores costarum; Multifidus; Rotatores, and Sacrospinalis.

bowling	rolling ball
ball games	tossing, catching, hitting
darts	throwing
croquet, golf	swinging and hitting
canoeing	paddling
fencing	thrusting
swimming	sidestroke
jacks	grabbing jacks
gardening	hoeing, shoveling, spading

38. Thorax: Inspiration

    Muscles involved—Diaphragm; External intercostals; Serratus posterior; Serratus superior; Scalenus anterior; Scalenus medius; Scalenus posterior; Sternocleidomastoideus, and Platysma.

exercise	to produce labored respiration
drinking	through a straw

39. Thorax: Expiration

    Muscles involved—Internal intercostals; Serratus posterior; Serratus inferior; Rectus abdominis; Transversus abdominis; External oblique, and Internal oblique.

exercise	to produce labored respiration
balloon	blowing up balloons

40. Abdomen

Muscles involved—Rectus abdominis; Internal oblique; External oblique; Transversus abdominis.

'curl'	lying on back, hands resting on thighs, slowly raising head and back
'uncurl'	reverse, use arms for partial support

41. Thigh: Flexion

Muscles involved—Iliacus; Psoas major; Sartorius; Rectus femoris; Pectineus; Cracilius; Adductor magnus; Adductor longus, Adductor brevis, and Tensor facialata.

ping pong	walking
weaving	lifting thigh to treadle
bicycle	peddling
ceramics	foot-powered potter's wheel
gardening	stooping
swimming	diving, frog, kick, scissors
bowling	walking, release ball
horseshoes	posting
shuffleboard	pushing puck
fencing	thrusting
dancing	all
skating	gliding
baseball	batting, running, kicking
golf	walking
hop scotch	hopping
skating	as in walking
tumbling	somersaults

42. Thigh: Extension

Muscles involved—Gluteus maximus; Biceps femoris; Semitendinosis; Semimembranosis, and Adductor magnus.

weaving	pushing down treadle
ping pong	quick foot movements
pottery	foot-powered potter's wheel
woodwork	bicycle saw
swimming	scissors kick, flutter kick
bowling	lunge to throw ball
gardening	pushing wheelbarrow
scooter	pushing to make it go
dancing	dip, quick movements
roller skating	pushing to roll or slide
ball games	running or jumping
golf	walking, swinging

Social and Behavioral Factors in Program Content

43. Thigh: Abduction

    Muscles involved—Gluteus medius; Gluteus minimus; Piriformis; Sartorius; Gemellus inferior; Gemellus superior; Obturator internus, and Tensor fascia lata.

weaving	reaching for pedals
swimming	frog kick
dancing	lunges, kicks
rowing	bracing feet
hop scotch	jumping
ping pong	reaching
horseback riding	mounting
fencing	lunge
tennis	reaching to hit
exercise	sitting tailor fashion

44. Thigh: Adduction

    Muscles Involved—Quadratus femoris; Gracilis; Pectineus; Adductor magnus; Adductor longus; Adductor brevis, and Obturator externus.

gardening	stooping, spading
swimming	frog kick, backstroke, breaststroke
horseback riding	straddling, gripping
ping pong	moving legs
roller skating	crossing legs around turns
dancing	all
tennis	running, side-stepping
wrestling	body slam, holding with legs

45. Thigh: Outward Rotation

    Muscles involved—Quadratus femoris; Piriformis; Obturator externus; Obturator internus; Gemellus superior, and Gemellus inferior.

weaving	treadling
pottery	kick wheel
fencing	lunge
golf	swinging
ball games	batting, pivoting
diving	race position

46. Thigh: Inward Rotation

    Muscles involved—Gluteus minimus.

wrestling	any hold
soccer	kicking

horseback riding	posting
basketball	pivoting
woodwork	planing
golf	putting

47. Leg: Flexion

    Muscles involved–Sartorius; Gracilis; Semimembranosis; Semitendonosis; Popliteus; Biceps femoris; Gastrocnemius, and Plantaris.

pottery	treadling on wheel
track	running and jumping
baseball	catching, running
basketball	running, springing
golf	swinging and walking
swimming	scissors kick, frog kick, diving
tumbling	somersaults
fencing	lunging
dancing	all
hiking	over hilly ground
gardening	stooping, weeding

48. Leg: Inward Rotation

    Muscles involved–Sartorius; Semimembranosis; Semitendinosis; and Popliteus.

dancing	Charleston
track	running

49. Leg: Extension

    Muscles involved–Rectus femoris; Vastus lateralis; Vastus medialis, and Vastus intermedius.

gardening	spading, pushing wheelbarrow
weaving	treadling
dancing	dips
football	kicking
fencing	lunge
golf	swinging, walking
cycling	pedaling
swimming	scissors and frog kick
bowling	stride
ice skating	skating backwards

50. Leg: Outward Rotation

    Muscles involved–Biceps Femoris.

Social and Behavioral Factors in Program Content

dancing	ballet
swimming	diving
ice skating	spread eagle
cycling	pedaling

51. Ankle and Foot: Dorsal Flexion

   Muscles involved—Tibialis anterior; Peroneus tertius; Extensor digitorum longus, and Extensor hallicus longus.

piano	working pedals
cycling	pedals
roller skating	raising skates from floor
walking	up steep grades
swimming	kicking
skipping rope	landing on toes
rowing	bracing feet
football	running and kicking
bowling	approach and ball release
tennis	running and jumping

52. Ankle and Foot: Plantar Flexion

   Muscles involved—Tibialis posterior; Soleus; Gastrocnemius; Peroneus longus; Peroneus brevis; Plantaris; Flexor digitorum longus, and Flexor hallicus longus.

cycling	pedals
gardening	stooping
weaving	treadles
diving	springing from board on toes
swimming	kicking
running	on toes
discus	rising on toes in approach
jumping	approach and land on toes
ball games	running, jumping, and shooting
trampolene	landing on toes
piano playing	pedals

53. Ankle and Foot: Eversion

   Muscles involved—Peroneus tertius; Peroneus longus; and Peroneus brevis.

pottery	kicking wheel
weaving	pedaling
baseball	batting and pitching
dancing	Charleston

54. Ankle and Foot: Inversion

Muscles involved—Tibialis anterior; Tibialis posterior; Extensor hallicus longus; Gastrocnemius; Flexor digitorum longus, and Flexor hallicus longus.

golf	stance when swinging
pottery	kicking wheel
soccer	kicking ball with side of foot
weaving	moving feet from treadle to treadle

In addition to concern for indications and contraindications with muscle and joint movement, the therapeutic recreation specialist must also be concerned with other sensory-motor factors which influence participation.

In some settings a classification system regarding activity involvement as a consequence of heart disease is used. The classification is decided upon as a result of the disease and refers to *functional* capacity or limitation imposed upon the patient or client because of cardiac impairment. There is also a prognositic classification which indicates activity restrictions necessary to prevent further impairment. The term "ordinary physical activity" used in the classification system, refers to the activity pattern prior to the onset of manifest cardiac disease. The system was developed by the American Heart Association and often used by vocational counselors in assessing employment capacity after treatment.

Post Cardiac Disease Classification System

FUNCTIONAL CAPACITY

Classification	Description
I	No limitation of physical activity; ordinary physical activity causes no discomfort.
II	Slight limitation of physical activity; ordinary physical activity causes discomfort.
III	Marked limitation of physical activity; discomfort caused by less than ordinary physical activity.
IV	Unable to carry on any physical activity without discomfort.

PREVENTIVE CLASSIFICATION

Classification	Description
A	Activity need not be restricted.
B	Ordinary physical activity need not be restricted, but unusually severe or competitive efforts should be avoided.
C	Ordinary physical activity should be moderately restricted; strenuous habitual efforts should be avoided.

Social and Behavioral Factors in Program Content

D   Ordinary physical activity should be markedly restricted.
E   Should be at complete rest, confined to bed or chair.

With respect to other conditions, there have been a variety of clinical classifications in use over the years. Many of these are modified with respect to new information, public taste, and change in attitude. For example, in relation to mental retardation, a medical classification was in vogue for a long time which used the terms idiot, imbecile, moron. Today a different system is used— profoundly retarded, severely retarded, moderately retarded, mildly retarded, slow learner. (Further discussion of this topic is presented in the following section on the Cognitive Domain.) For a long while a clinical classification for pulmonary tuberculosis was used when this disease was prominent and widespread. This latter classification provided information regarding physical and social participation because of the contagion factors.

Pulmonary Tuberculosis Clinical Classification (modified)

CLINICAL STATUS

Inactive No symptoms of tuberculous origin, repeatedly negative by microscopic examination and other clinical tests; xray reveals lesions to be stable, slow shrinkage, no cavitation; period of inactivity beyond 6 months is —
    Inactive _____ months.

Active Symptoms commonly present, clinical tests almost always indicate tubercle bacilli; xray usually reveals progressive or retrogressive lesions; period of activity if known is stated —
    Active _____ months (years).

Improved
Unimproved This designation will sometimes be used after "Active" on repeated examination.

Undetermined A temporary designation when activity of disease is not clear or has not been adequately determined.

ACTIVITY STATUS

I Bed rest; varying from strict immobilization to bathroom privileges.
II Semi-ambulatory; modified bed rest, meals in common dining room, mass entertainment, and other activities gradually reaching a total period of four hours out of bed each day.
III Ambulatory; further progression of activity such as planned walks, craft shop, classes, and club meetings.
IV Ordinary living conditions; return to former activity pattern consistent with limitations.

Depending upon the setting for service, the Specialist will find the classification system in use of help in understanding the effect of pathology upon patient or client's physical activity involvement in the program. This becomes extremely important with regard to goal-oriented programs. Some other usual classifications include: *Diabetes*—1. well regulated by diet alone; 2. regulated by diet and insulin, 3. regulated by diet and insulin but does not abide by requirements, 4. severe condition, well regulated diet and insulin, unstabilized condition subject to shock or coma. *Arthritis*—1. pain and stiffness, not limited; 2. pain and stiffness lowers activity involvement; 3. pain and stiffness curtails activity involvement; 4. pain and stiffness precludes or severely limits activity involvement. If the Specialist is employed in a setting in which large numbers of patients or clients are limited in activity participation because of physical pathology, a single classification system which facilitates communication of this type of information will prove beneficial. In the final section of this chapter information is given which has application toward this objective.

Cognitive Domain

Perhaps as a consequence of industrialization or the historical precedence of the anatomist, psychologists through the ages have been attempting to develop a structure for the mind. This "mapping" of the mind has taken many

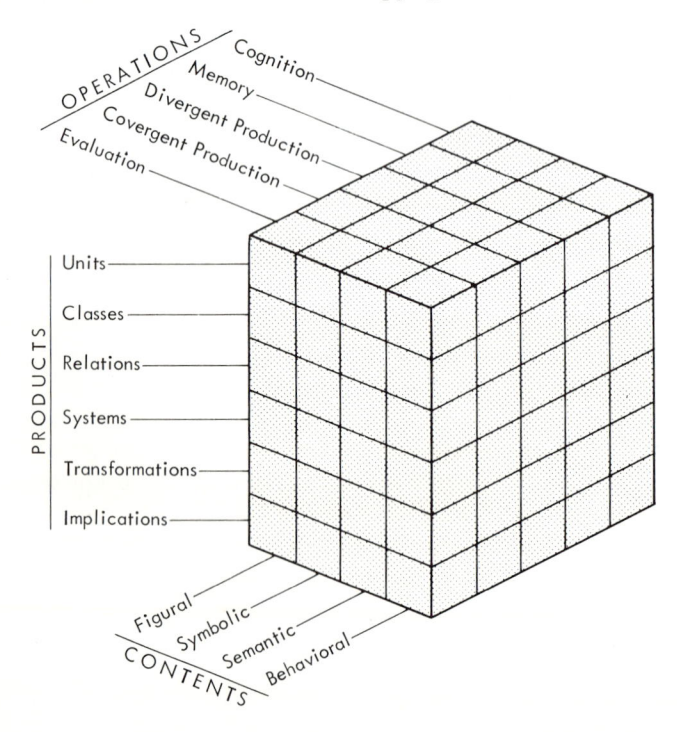

THE STRUCTURE OF INTELLECT (Guilford and Hoepfner).
Reprinted by permission of the authors.

forms, and there is no universal agreement as there is in dealing with the sensory-motor domain. In fact, the "mind" is divided into two domains—the cognitive domain, which concerns intellectual functioning, and the affective domain, which concerns emotions.

There are many models in the literature for the *cognitive* domain. One major model which tends to offer a parallel to the physical structure of the sensory-motor domain is the model proposed by Guilford and his associates over the past two decades.[4]

Guilford's model for "The Structure of Intellect" is based on the notion that the first task of intellect is to discriminate information. Information may be presented to or recalled by the individual in a number of forms which Guilford has grouped and labeled as *content*. In the theoretical parallel with the sensory-motor domain, in which solids and fluids are processed by the body systems, informational content is the substance which the intellect processes. There are four groups of content according to Guilford:

> *Figural Content*—concrete forms and images that may be auditory, visual, kinetic, or a combination, and have meaning in themselves;
> *Symbolic Content*—signs and symbols such as letters or musical notation or numbers, which have no significance in themselves, but stand for other things;
> *Semantic Content*—meanings to which words are attached, and which are used in thinking and communication;
> *Behavioral Content*—nonverbal information derived from observation of human interaction, such as attitudes, moods, intentions, and the like.

Although the sensory-motor domain processes solids and fluids through the processes of digestion, osmosis, circulation, and the like, the intellect processes informational content through a complex system which Guilford calls *operations*.

In his model, Guilford refers to the first operation as *cognition*—the immediate discovery, or awareness, rediscovery, or recognition of information. Cognition is the sensitivity of the intellect to informational stimuli. *Memory* is the process that stores and retrieves information. Information is stored with some degree of availability, and is retrieved based upon the cues with which it was learned. *Evaluation* is the operation or process that is concerned with a variety of judgments concerning the correctness, suitability, adequacy, desirability, consistency, and so forth of information. Finally, *divergent production* and *convergent production* are two processing operations that are concerned with generation of information from given information. Divergent production is

---

[4] J. P. Guilford, *The Nature of Human Intelligence* (Toronto: McGraw-Hill Book Co., 1967); and J. P. Guilford and R. Hoepfner, *The Analysis of Intelligence* (Toronto: McGraw-Hill Book Co., 1971); M. Garrison (Ed.) *Cognitive Models and Development in Mental Retardation*, Monograph Supplement to the American Journal of Mental Deficiency, 70(4), 1966.

concerned with variety and quantity of output, while convergent production is concerned with the best or unique solutions.

As in the sensory-motor domain, in which the body processes result in a variety of products such as tissue, bone, chemicals, waste products, and others, the intellectual operations result in *products*—new forms of information. Guilford has referred to these as *units, classes, relations, systems, transformations,* and *implications.* Thus, for example, a product would be a unit of information, a class of information, or a transformation of information.

Although Guilford's model is not universally accepted, there are close parallels in the work of Piaget and a number of psychologists, and since the time of Dewey, theoretical attempts to explain how we think have been published. Guilford's model has been modified a number of times, and will probably continue to be modified as more is learned about the brain and behavior. Its value in therapeutic recreation service is that it enables one to understand impairment in intellectual functioning in a more concrete fashion than just the notion of mental retardation, or the vague generalizations associated with "low IQ." It offers, as in the case of the sensory-motor domain, an opportunity to understand specific behavioral limitations. Just as there may be a disturbance in strength or balance, digestion or circulation, or some other physical process, there may be an intellectual impairment in evaluation, cognition, filtering, convergent production, and the like. Just as a physician uses a number of testing methods to determine impairment in a muscle or joint, a psychologist can test for impairment in intellect with respect to Guilford's model. Activities that rely heavily on convergent production, for example, would not be included in a patient or client's program if it is known that he has an impairment in this intellectual operation. Similarly, if the patient or client has considerable difficulty with the production of "classes" or "relations," an activity that calls for these kinds of results would not be included in his programs.

In 1961, the American Association on Mental Deficiency published a monograph entitled *A Manual on Terminology and Classification in Mental Retardation*. This manual indicated that mental retardation was not only a condition which originated during the developmental period and resulted in subaverage general intellectual functioning, but there was also impairment in "adaptive behavior" as a consequence. Leland and a team of AAMD psychologists in the United States devised a scale for classifying adaptive behavior associated with impaired cognition.

General Adaptive Behavior Levels (modified)

Level	Description
I	Capable of effective social and economic functioning in *low-demand competitive environment*; needs support and supervision in management of personal affairs.

II	Capable of effective social and economic functioning in a *partially competitive environment*; needs continuing support and supervision in the management of personal affairs.
III	Capable of limited social and economic functioning in a *noncompetitive or sheltered environment*; needs general control and support in personal affairs.
IV	Capable of responding to the *simplest of environmental stimuli* and interpersonal relationships; needs nursing supervision for maintenance and help in routines of daily living.
V	Gross physical impairment; requires continuous medical-nursing care for survival.

Gunzberg in England has developed a number of scales to chart and assess progress in relation to cognitive impairment and treatment or training. He indicates that assessment should be examined with regard to self-help, communication, vocation, and socialization. Similarly, Spier in The Netherlands has advocated that cognitive impairment must be looked at with regard to behavior in more than 'just' intellectual functioning. Considerable research on the cognitive domain continues throughout the world today in an attempt to understand this domain with the specificity in which we now understand the sensory-motor domain. Applying this same type of understanding to the affective domain is not possible at this time.

Affective Domain

Work on the affective domain seems to differ with each school of psychology. If we use Guilford's classifications for information, we find that some schools of psychology are primarily concerned with behavioral information and their models only concern this type of information, while another school is primarily concerned with figural information. Psychoanalysis appears to be primarily concerned with symbolic information, and the Rogerians with semantic information. Each school of thought has promulgated different processes or operations. Jung, for example, proposed such operations as compensation, opposition, unification, transcendence, and symbolization. Fromm speaks of reception, exploiting, hoarding, marketing, producing. Freud wrote about mental mechanisms or defense mechanisms, indicating that there were more than two dozen of these, including association, catharsis, displacement, identification, rationalization, suppression, transference, regression, and the like. Sullivan referred to operations as dynamisms and proposed a different set. Other, more contemporary clinical theoreticians have additional models. As in the case of cognitive operations, there can be impairment in affective operations. When this occurs, a person is said to be "fixated" and thus all his behavior is dominated by the impaired process or operation. The following illustrates this situation.

Mr. J. doesn't often become involved in activity, but when he does, he looks to the recreation leader for direction. He shows no initiative. When asked if he likes or dislikes something, Mr. J. does not venture an opinion. He hesitates to try anything new—he invariably predicts that he will be unable to do what's involved. He appears to have no confidence in himself. He constantly seeks reassurance that the leader and everyone else likes him. Words don't seem to reassure him enough, for he actually "hangs on" to the leader. He usually will do what the leader asks him to do, and responds in a polite, optimistic fashion, almost friendly. Mr. J. makes a strong effort to give the impression that he wants to comply with the leader's wishes but states in a number of ways that he is helpless, can do nothing of any value alone, and that he can't act without direction. One gets the impression that although Mr. J. says yes, he would like to say no, but can't bring himself to do so.

He tells you his doctor is wonderful, and is going to make him well. He knows that all he has to do is follow the doctor's orders, and sees this as his only responsibility in the process. Mr. J. seems to respond in the same way to both men and women. He demonstrates no preference for one or the other. He makes friends with anyone that will have him, and he refrains from being critical of anyone. He doesn't discriminate between feeling friendship and merely going through the motions of friendly behavior. Mr. J. becomes very anxious during card games when he has to decide what card to play, or during other games when it is up to him to move a token on the board. Sometimes he becomes so upset he leaves the game. He enjoys listening to music, watching motion pictures, television viewing, and any other solitary activity in which all he does is sit and receive. He has enormous difficulty in arts and crafts, unless given detailed instructions, and when left alone, rarely finishes what he starts. He likes parties best, especially when refreshments are served. Food seems to mean a lot to Mr. J. He responds well to motherly volunteers and praises them for the fine work they do, particularly the volunteers who serve food or give out candy and cigarettes. On the whole, Mr. J. creates little or no problem for the recreation leader. He is easily pleased, and can always be used when an extra pair of hands are needed. He is happy to respond to the leader's request to move chairs or carry a message. Volunteers observe that Mr. J. is "so pleasant and so appreciative" of the work volunteers do. With each day of hospitalization, Mr. J. seems to become sicker. He appears more passive, more dependent, and on occasion stays in bed all day, eating only when he is hand-fed. On visiting day, Mr. J.'s cousin remarked to the recreation leader, "What a pity that this should happen to him. He never did any harm. He's such a nice guy!"

In contrast to Mr. J., who appears to function as a "sponge," or "receiver," is the following example.

Mr. G. creates a great many problems for the recreation leader. He doesn't care about anyone else and boasts that he can do just about anything. He uses staff, volunteers, and other patients for his own ends. He has a number of followers among the other patients. If he can "call the shots" he and his followers will enter into any activity. He does poorly in arts and crafts, and when he wants a certain item, rather than make it himself, he steals it from one of his followers, or in other instances, seduces another person into giving it to him. At parties, when refreshments are served, Mr. G. has a "boarding-house reach." He pushes his way into organized groups, and tries to take over. He won't bother with isolates. He seems to delight in taking other people's property, including their friends. He lacks originality. He is quick to seize someone else's ideas, professing that these are his. He is bright and shows considerable initiative. He acts impulsively, and when frustrated, he becomes belligerent. Mr. G. has a quick, sarcastic, and cynical tongue. He dominates his followers, and is envious and jealous of others. He demands things from the recreation leader, and never seems to be satisfied with the activities offered. He expresses considerable dissatisfaction with the way the recreation specialist and other members of the staff "run things around here." For the most part, Mr. G. makes no differentiation between men and women. He recently got into an argument with a woman staff member, which ended with his punching her. The only differentiation Mr. G. seems to make is between those who have authority and power to give and those who haven't.

A third example of an impairment in affective processing or operations is in the following material.

> Miss R. is a challenge to the recreation leader. She is apparently unimaginative and behaves in a lethargic manner. When she is invited to join an activity she appears cautious, reserved, and suspicious of the recreation leader's motives. It is difficult to get a response from her. She doesn't laugh or smile often, nor does she express anger. She seems to be more interested in things than people. She refuses square dancing, dramatics, any team sport, bridge, and also refuses to help decorate for a party. She does like crafts if she is allowed to sit and work alone, and permitted to keep what she makes. She chooses the most uncomfortable chairs, preferably those that are in the corner of a room. She is neat and orderly about what she does. Miss R. becomes anxious when something is lost, or the score in a game is not kept accurately, or a game is not played exactly according to the rules. She prefers tether ball to table tennis. In one instance, she participated in a game where the purpose was to find certain objects. When the leader stopped the game before all the objects were found Miss R. became obviously disturbed and refused to leave the room until all the objects were found. Miss R. becomes upset when anyone flicks ashes on the floor or if a cup of coffee is accidently spilled. She has been called a "pig" by the volunteers. They state that if they don't watch her she takes much more than her share. She has been seen stuffing cookies and cake into her mouth with one hand, her cheeks bulging, and taking more from the plate with the other hand at the same time. Miss R. is meticulous about her hair, constantly smoothing it down, and much

concerned with the orderliness of her clothing. She uses the bathroom frequently to wash her hands—sometimes before, during, and after each activity. She sometimes works a jig-saw puzzle. Before beginning, she carefully counts all the pieces to see if they correspond to the number printed on the box. Miss R. becomes anxious if she has to leave before finishing the puzzle. Even when there is lots of time, she works at the puzzle incessantly until it is finished. She takes things although she has no apparent use for them. When allowed to use certain equipment, she considers it her property and becomes quite possessive of it. She becomes anxious if a session doesn't begin or end on time, and hounds the recreation leader about this. She often volunteers to straighten up the supply closet. On one occasion, when the recreation leader could not permit Miss R. to take a phonograph record back to her room, she smashed the record.

These three examples indicate impairment in operations which might be referred to as "receiving," "taking," and "keeping." The following material is illustrative of the affective process associated with "getting." On the whole, impairments in this affective operation appear to result in a lack of direction and a seeming "living from day to day." There is an aimlessness in behavior, and a dislike for being alone. Other behaviors include a lack of tact, nondiscrimination, and indifference. There is a tendency to be overactive.

At a recreation activity, Mr. H. and Miss S. challenge the male recreation leader to a duel at chess, table tennis, bowling, blackjack, or any activity in which there is a chance to beat the leader. Mr. H. seems constantly compelled to prove his capability and manliness. He has great difficulty getting along with the female recreation leader and with women in general. At dances Mr. H. either withdraws into a corner or goes to the other extreme and plays the part of a Don Juan with all the women in the room. Mr. H. prefers stag activities though and often boasts of his masculine prowess. He is eager to try his hand at boxing with the male recreation leader, but wrestling, tumbling, and gymnastics are taboo as far as he's concerned, because he states that he doesn't like to touch other men. Miss M. ignores the female recreation leader and never offers to compete with her. Miss M. appears uncomfortable at dances. She prefers to dance with other women. She avoids physical contact with men, and becomes obviously more anxious when it is unavoidable. However, she eagerly involves herself in activity where there may be physical contact with other women.

Mr. O. and Miss F., on the other hand, are more responsive to the female recreation leader than to the male recreation leader. Both of them like to play checkers and table tennis with the female recreation leader. They both enjoy dances and are quite skilled. Mr. O. does an excellent job at party decorations, and Miss F. is quite a hand with refreshments. Mr. O. tends to choose activities which involve more women than men. Miss F. is very ladylike, and gets along well with other women. She doesn't like to

Social and Behavioral Factors in Program Content 207

dance, but since she knows how, she does allow the recreation leader to dance with her.

In contrast, Mr. A. and Miss W. don't seem to get along with anybody. They lack social skills, and are verbally aggressive to both male and female recreation leaders. They usually refuse to enter into any activity. They often stand scowling on the fringes of an activity. Mr. A. picks fights with other participants, and Miss W. often gets angry and breaks things. Once in a while Mr. A. does get involved in an activity, but before long he becomes demanding and abusive. Miss W. usually disregards the rules of a game when she gets involved, and "makes no bones" about cheating. Both of them usually take what they want, bully others, and show no remorse for their behavior.

Finally, there are Mr. N. and Miss M., who try to please. They are the first ones to respond to anything the recreation leader suggests. Others refer to them as the "personality kids." At a Mexican Night Party, Miss M. was the most Mexican; at a carnival night, Mr. N. was the most "carnival." Both seem carefree and are consistently pleasant-mannered. They get along with men, women, dogs, fish, and any living thing around. There is not an activity which they won't enter into, so long as it involves others. When Mr. N. is alone he becomes very restless. If another person is looking for a listener Mr. N. will listen; if a talker is needed, he will talk, if someone wants followers, he will follow; if a number of persons need a leader, he will try to lead. He is perfectly adaptable. If Miss M. is watching television and it bothers someone, she will turn it off. If she is playing the piano and someone doesn't like what she is playing she will stop, and try to play what they want to hear, even if she doesn't know the piece. Mr. N. and Miss M. both have many skills and know how to do many things. They have numerous friends and acquaintances, they are name-droppers, and know all the best places to go. Mr. N. is a member of Rotary and the JCC. Miss M. is a member of the Junior League and the Federation of Women's Clubs. They both have a large reservoir of funny stories and witty sayings. If the recreation leader expresses any displeasure with their behavior, they can change it on the spot. Whatever kind of behavior the leader is buying, they have it to sell. They behave one way in one situation, and an entirely different fashion in other situations. At a staff meeting, it became apparent that the behavior of Mr. N. and Miss M. reflects whatever the person in charge considers appropriate behavior.

What are the products of these affective operations? General agreement would be that they are emotion, feeling, affect, sentiment, mood, passion, and the like. These products are described with such words as anxiety, love, fear, joy, despair, chagrin, elation, misery, affection, ambivalence, and hundreds of others. Thus it becomes apparent to the therapeutic recreation specialist that discussion and action concerning affective impairment will differ from setting to setting, dependent upon the orientation of the psychiatrists and psychologists in that setting. The following are some common terms used in psychiatric settings to describe behavioral products of the affective domain, with some examples of resultant behavior, and approaches that might be taken.

agitation	restlessness, fear, and excitement, pacing the floor, wringing the hands, rubbing and picking at the skin, worries and complaints.
anxiety	strong feelings of uncertainty and fear; sometimes the word "apprehension" is used to indicate the same behavior.
apathy	feelings of indifference.
assaultive	striking out or fighting with others.
belligerent	arguing and threatening others; appears to be ready to start a fight.
bizarre	strange behavior, strange dress, or strange personal appearance.
confabulation	inability to remember the truth, so invents a story about a past event.
depression	strong feelings of sadness.
disoriented	not knowing where he is, what day it is, or who he is.
distractibility	noticing every sound or motion in the immediate vicinity.
elation	great happiness or pleasure without apparent cause.
hyperactive	overly active.
hoarding	collecting and hiding of unnecessary things such as paper, string, etc.
illusion	seeing or hearing something which he thinks is something else.
incoherent	jumbled speech which cannot be understood by others.
instability	rapid mood changes without apparent cause.
mute	does not speak.
negativism	doing the opposite of what is expected.
panic	strongest, worst kind of fear.
preoccupation	lost deep in thought.
seclusive	staying away from others, keeping to oneself.
stupor	seems unconscious.
suggestible	easily influenced by words and acts of others.

As in the case of the sensory-motor domain (with respect to physical limitations and activity involvement), the therapeutic recreation specialist is primarily interested in those aspects of the cognitive and affective domain which are not impaired and which will allow successful participation. However, and particularly with regard to the affective domain, popular recreative activity is often used to assist in treatment of a patient or client with affective limitations, particularly in Western society. Explanation of some of these approaches will be found in the literature.

A final aspect of recreation with regard to the affective domain should be mentioned in passing. This is the concept of "pathological play." Any activity that is inherently destructive to life is pathological—an example is "Russian

Social and Behavioral Factors in Program Content 209

roulette," a game in which a single cartridge is put into the magazine of a revolver and the magazine is spun so the players do not know where the cartridge is. The players put the gun to their heads (one person at a time), betting that they will survive. A similar pathological activity is played by young children who jump across roofs of buildings, or hang onto the moving undercarriages of elevators. These latter activities go under the name of *"chicken."* Other, equally destructive activities could be cited. However, there are a number of seemingly innocent activities that are not pathological in themselves, but are pathological when viewed in the context of a participant's life situation. They may not be overtly physically destructive to an individual, but they are psychologically pathological in that they are destructive to his personality.[5]

Now that we have briefly examined aspects of the three behavioral domains, we are ready to consider the final element in the activity matrix.

Abilities And Skills Required For Participation

Participation in any activity requires the utilization of a variety of abilities and skills. However, each activity requires a specific combination or set of abilities and skills, and thus one element of any given activity is the special character of the abilities and skills a person must possess in order to engage in the activity. Theoretically, the activity itself specifies which abilities and skills a person must have; for example, the ability to throw a ball, the ability to remember which cards have been played, and the ability to identify with a character in a play. Because all activity requires the utilization of some behavioral ability and varying degrees of skill, it is erroneous to classify an activity as "not active" or "passive." Watching television, for example, requires the ability to see, to hold oneself in a position to view the screen and a host of other abilities in the cognitive and affective domains.

For ease of studying human abilities and skills, scholars have classified these into behavioral domains. Participation in any activity requires the utilization of abilities and skills in *all* three domains; however, some activities require *more* skill in one domain and *lesser* skill utilization of the other two domains; some activities require skill in two domains and *lesser* utilization of the third domain. Some activities require considerable interaction of abilities and skills in all three domains.

With regard to recreative activity, it is possible to classify activity in relation to the specification of abilities and skills grouped by behavioral domain. An even more exacting classification can be undertaken if activities are grouped with respect to which domain is predominant; that is, the primary focus of the activity: intellect, emotion, or movement. (Sensory perception is assumed in all participation.)

The following offers examples and illustrates a method for coding

[5] Paul Haun, "Pathological Play," *Recreation: A Medical Viewpoint* ed. E. M. Avedon and F. B. Arje (New York: Teachers College Press, 1965), p. 22.

activities for programming or research purposes using this classification scheme. The code utilizes ten items:

- A an activity that requires predominantly cognitive skills.

    Example: crossword puzzle. Although a participant needs such additional abilities from the other two domains as the ability to grasp a pencil and write in the squares, and some ability to tolerate frustration when he cannot recall the correct response, the focus of the activity is upon such intellectual skills as memory and convergent production.

- B an activity that requires predominantly affective skills.

    Example: viewing a play. Although a participant needs such additional abilities from the other two domains as the ability to remain erect in a theater seat for a period of time and the ability to be aware of the meaning of the plot, the focus of the activity is upon such affective skills as identification, empathy, and the like.

- AB an activity that requires predominantly cognitive skills, but also relies upon affective abilities.

    Example: a board game—Chinese Friends. Although a participant needs such abilities from the sensory-motor domain as vision and the ability to grasp and release a counter on the board, the focus of the activity is upon such intellectual skills as evaluation and convergent production. However, because each participant experiences a constant shift in status, the ability to control one's temper so cognitive abilities are not impeded is also important.

- BA an activity that requires predominantly affective abilities, but also relies upon cognitive abilities.

    Example: a "collecting hobby." Although a participant needs such manual skills as the hobby requires, the focus of the activity is upon such emotional abilities as appreciation, affection, and compulsiveness; however, such intellectual skills as cognition, evaluation, and memory are required for success in the activity.

- C an activity that requires predominantly sensory-motor abilities.

    Example: body-building. Although a participant needs such cognitive skills as evaluation and such affective abilities as egocentricity or narcissism, the focus of the activity is upon such sensory-motor abilities and skills as strength, flexibility, and grasp.

- CA an activity that requires predominantly sensory-motor abilities, but also relies upon cognitive abilities.

    Example: knitting. Although a participant needs such emotional skills as a degree of compulsiveness, the focus of the activity is on the flexibility of the fingers and arms and the ability to count, read instructions, and translate the instructions into patterns.

Social and Behavioral Factors in Program Content 211

CB   an activity that requires predominantly sensory-motor skills, but relies upon affective ability as well.

Example: horseback riding. Although a participant needs such cognitive skills as judgment, focus of the activity is upon the physical stamina to sit on the horse and the ability not to fear the horse, or the ability to demonstrate ego strength.

AC   an activity that requires predominantly cognitive ability, but also relies upon sensory-motor ability.

Example: constructing a stereo system from a kit. Although a participant needs such affective ability as patience, the focus of the activity is upon reading blueprints, judging which wires are to be joined, and many other similar evaluations. However, success is also determined by one's ability in the sensory-motor domain such as grasping ability, fine muscle coordination, steadiness, and the like.

BC   an activity that requires predominantly affective abilities, but also relies upon sensory-motor ability.

Example: listening to a concert. Although the participant needs such intellectual ability as to be able to understand the intricacies of orchestration, the focus of the activity is upon appreciation, imagination, and the crucial ability to hear the music.

ABC an activity in which apparently no one behavioral domain is predominant.

Example: playing a musical instrument. The participant needs sufficient motor ability to play, sufficient cognitive ability to read musical notations and translate the symbols into action, and sufficient affective ability to give the resultant sound color, warmth, and feeling.

Using this classification scheme, it becomes possible for a therapeutic recreation specialist to label activities in a program with respect to indications and counterindications for various perspective participants. It is also a device that can be used for supervising personnel with less experience and education, as well as volunteers. Finally, it may be used as a system of classification in research. It must be remembered, however, that it is only a theoretical tool, and as such has many limitations.

The following selected references offer examples of the types of material concerning program content that appear in the literature. Certain documents are specific to one disorder, while others are concerned with a group of disorders. Some documents include only "how-to" information, while others examine certain clinical ramifications of a popular recreative activity. It is interesting to note the range of document sources that publish information about therapeutic recreation service, as indicated previously by Martin in Chapter 4.

Program Content. Bibliographic Examples

Adams, R. C., A. Daniel, and L. Rullman, *Games, Sports and Exercises for the Physically Handicapped.* Philadelphia: Lea & Febiger, 1972.

Adatto, C., "On Play and the Psychopathology of Golf," *Journal of the American Psychoanalytic Association,* XII, No. 4 (1964), 826-41.

American Academy of Pediatrics—Committee on Children with Handicaps, "The Epileptic Child and Competitive School Athletics," *Pediatrics,* XLII, No. 4 (1968), 700-702.

Archer, J., "Basketball Comes to Hospital Patients," *Recreation,* XLVII, No. 4 (1954), 227.

Barclay, D., "Emotional Stakes in Playing Games," *New York Times Magazine,* August 7, 1955, 43.

Bauer, D., "Big-Ten Football, Wheelchair Style," *Recreation,* LII, No. 11 (1959), 386-87.

Beisser, A., *The Madness in Sports.* New York: Appleton-Century-Crofts, 1967.

Beresford, A., "Team Games and Recreation in Mental Hospitals," *Nursing Mirror,* CLXXX, November 27, 1959, 5-7.

Bergler, E., *The Psychology of Gambling.* New York: Hill and Wang, 1957.

Bevans, J. E., "Development of a Recreational Music Program at Perkins School for the Blind," *International Journal for Education of the Blind,* XIV, No. 3 (1965), 72-76.

Blau, L., "Appliances and Remedial Games," *American Journal of Physical Medicine,* XXXIV, No. 8 (1955), 498-510.

Boeshart, L. K., "Remedial Games in Treatment of Physical Disability," *American Journal of Occupational Therapy,* V, No. 3 (1951), 47-48.

Boyd, N., *Hospital and Bedside Games,* Chicago: H. T. Fitzsimmons Co., Inc., 1919; rev., 1945.

Braaten, J., and I. Lee, *Swimming Program for the Trainable Retarded—Guide #1: Organization and Administration of the Program,* Toronto: Canadian Association of the Mentally Retarded, n.d., 16 pp.

Brachman, D. S., "Observation on the Cardiac Unit of a Fresh-Air Camp: On the Use or Avoidance of Sports," *Journal of Aviation Medicine,* III, No. 6 (1932), 109-15.

Brown, M. E., "Ten Motion Games For Fun and Therapy," *American Journal of Nursing,* LVI, No. 1 (1956), 44-48.

———, "Therapy for the Orthopedically Exceptional: An Analysis of Twenty-five Games," *American Journal of Occupational Therapy,* XXIV, No. 8 (1945), 171-78.

Brown, R. L., and O. L. McBain, "Social Activities for Educable Mentally Retarded High School and Post High School People," *Journal of Psychiatric Nursing,* III, No. 2 (1965), 133-37.

Buell, C. E., *Active Games for the Blind.* Ann Arbor, Michigan: Edwards Brothers, 1947.

———, *Sports for the Blind.* Ann Arbor, Michigan: Edwards Brothers, 1947.

Carlson, G., and D. Ginglend, *Play Activities for the Mentally Retarded Child.* New York: Abingdon Press, 1961, pp. 64-93.

Carr, A. C., "A Therapeutic Recreation Program For Children with Spina Bifida and Myelomeningocele," *Comprehensive Care of the Child with Spina Bifida Manifesta,* C. A. Swinyard, ed., New York: New York University Medical Center, 1966, pp. 131-33.

Carroccio, D. F., and L. F. Quattlebaum, "An Elementary Technique for Manipulation of Participation in Ward Dances at a Neuropsychiatric Hospital," *Journal of Music Therapy,* VI, No. 4 (1969), 108-109.

Chapman, F. M., *Recreation Activities for the Handicapped.* New York: Ronald Press, 1960, pp. 235-76.

Colby, K. M., "Gentlemen, The Queen!", *Psychoanalytic Review,* XL (1953), 144-48.

Danning, E., "The Value of Chess to the Quadriplegic Patient," *Recreation for the Ill and Handicapped* (October 1957).

Delany, E. "Assignment: Games For The Patient," *Recreation,* LIV, No. 1 (1961), 26-29.

Fell, J. H., "Producing a Show with Mentally Subnormal Patients," *Nursing Mirror,* CXXI, No. 3 (1965), 335-36.

Fox, S. S., "Games for Handicapped Children," *Recreation,* XLIV, No. 5 (1950), 93-94.

Frankel, L., and G. Frankel, *Muscle-Building Games.* New York: Sterling Publishing Corp., 1964.

Ginglend, D. R., and W. E. Stiles, *Music Activities for Retarded Children—A Handbook for Teachers and Parents.* Nashville, Tenn.: Abingdon Press, 1965, 140 pp.

Gray, P. E., "Therapeutic Recreation Service For the Chronic Brain Syndrome Patient in a Home and Hospital for the Aged," *Recreation in Treatment Centers,* V (1966), 12-14.

Gump, P. V., and B. Sutton-Smith, "The "It" Role in Children's Games," *The Group,* XVII (1955), 3-8.

Gump P. V., and M. Yueng-Hung, "Active Games for Physically Handicapped Children," *Physical Therapy Review,* XXXIV, No. 4 (1954), 4, 171.

Hyde, R. W., et al., "Effectiveness of Games in Mental Hospitals," *American Journal of Occupational Therapy,* XXVII, No. 8 (1948), 304-308.

Jokl, E., *Heart and Sport,* Springfield, Ill.: Charles C. Thomas, 1964.

Keffer, L., "Introduction to Swimming for the Deaf," *Outlook,* I, No. 1 (1969), 3.

Lindsay, Z., *Art for Spastics.* New York: Taplinger Publishing Co., 1966, 71 pp.

McKindree, O. J., "Bowling as a Psychiatric Adjunct," *Psychiatric Quarterly,* XXIV (1950), 303-307.

Mignoga, M., *The Selection of Games for Use in Cases of Cardiac Insufficiency.* New York: New York University, 1932.

Milita, E. J., "Modified Croquet and Golf for the Retarded," *Recreator,* Newsletter of the Woodbine State Colony, Woodbine, N. J., II, No. 4 (1966), 4.

Parker, D., *Teaching Swimming to the Disabled.* Toronto: Canadian Red Cross, 1972.

Prytherch, H., "Teaching the Severely Subnormal Adult to Swim," *Journal of Mental Subnormality,* XIV, No. 2 (1968), 62-69.

"Rally Around The Ball Pole," *Mental Hospitals,* X, No. 1 (1959), 23.

Raymond, E. B. "Bridge Anyone?", *Mental Hospitals,* XIV, No. 4 (1963), 226.

Richardson, U., *Games for the Handicapped.* London: C. Arthur Pearson, Ltd., 1956.

Roderman, C. R. "Let's Play Ball," *American Journal of Nursing,* XLIX, No. 4 (1949), 566-67.

Roger, G., and L. Thomas, "Toys, Games, and Apparatus for Children With Cerebral Palsy," *Physical Therapy Review,* XXIX, No. 1 (1949), 5.

Sapora, A. W., "Values of Sports and Games for the Ill and Handicapped," *Recreation for the Ill and Handicapped,* I, No. 4 (1957), 10.

Schattner, R., *Creative Dramatics for the Handicapped.* New York: John Day Co., 1967, 160 pp.

Slovenko, R., and J. A. Knight, *Motivations in Play, Games, and Sports.* Springfield, Ill.: Charles C. Thomas, 1967.

Stafford, G. T., *Sports for the Handicapped.* Englewood Cliffs, N.J.: Prentice-Hall, Inc., 1947.

Wisher, P. R., "Dance and the Deaf," *Journal of Health, Physical Education, and Recreation,* XL, No. 3 (1969), 81.

Wolf, G., *Adapted Sports, Games, and Square Dances--Recreation for the Handicapped.* Hartford: Connecticut Society for Crippled Children and Adults, Inc., 1962.

Wood, A., *Sound Games: Speech Correction for the Very Young.* New York: E. P. Dutton and Co., Inc., 1948.

Woodward, H. H., and W. C. Stone, "Art in Correctional Institutions," *Journal of Correctional Education,* XXII, No. 1 (1970), 5-6.

Wrightson, H. A., *Games and Exercises for Mental Defectives.* Cambridge, Mass.: Caustic-Claflin, Co., 1916.

12
Aspects of Professional Practice

The following material offers the student and the instructor an opportunity to examine aspects of professional practice in a number of situations. How a specialist responds in a given situation will vary, depending upon the many factors presented in previous chapters. Perhaps the major determinant is the individualized style of a particular specialist. Thus, each case should be viewed *not* as an ideal but rather as a prototype to which one may adapt his own original style.

Case #1

H. Stevenson, male, white, age 34, married, three children

Diagnosis: emphysema

Order: Report weekly observations of patient interaction with peers and authority figures. Prevent the patient from getting involved in arguments. Make known to patient what activities are available and permit him to engage in those he wishes to. Major intent is behavioral observation at this time. Report results of preliminary interview.

Summary of Preliminary Interview: Appointment was made through head nurse on patient's ward. Patient arrived ten minutes late. Stood at office door and looked around sheepishly. I looked up from my desk and asked if he were Mr. S., I invited him to come in and sit down. I asked if he knew who I was. He said that he had seen me around. I said I had talked with Dr. B.

yesterday, and she indicated that Mr. S. was interested in doing something while he was in the hospital. He said he wanted to do something. I asked if he had seen some of the scheduled activities in the hospital, since he had been here for a few weeks. He said that he had been very sick up until now, and could not leave his room. I discussed some of the scheduled activities with him and asked if any of these interested him. He replied, "Everything, and that's part of my trouble." I indicated that it was sometimes difficult to make a decision. He did not respond, but looked away. I asked him what he did for a living. He said, "I'm a salesman, but I'm more interested in radio and TV. When I was a kid, my brother and I used to fool around with a ham outfit; now he is working in TV. I can do a lot of the things at home, which you do here, like the woodwork and stuff. I'd like to work in your radio station, if that's possible." I told him that it might be possible, and asked him what he wanted to do in the station. He said that he'd like to announce music. I explained that it was a closed-circuit station, and only broadcasts inside the hospital. He said he understood that. I asked him what kind of music he was interested in. He said religious music, " . . .we can use some of that around here." He began to laugh. When he noticed I didn't, he stopped abruptly. We discussed some of the mechanics of preparing for a weekly program and I gave him a pamphlet about announcing. He said he was eager to read the pamphlet and would do that this afternoon. I said I would let Dr. B. know of our tentative plans, and also let the nurse know so a schedule could be arranged. He said, "She's rather young—but seems to know her job." I said, "Nurse H.?" and he responded, "No Dr. B.!" We both smiled, and I said I would see him on Monday.

Questions

1. Is the physician's request appropriate?
2. Does the specialist have enough information for the preliminary interview?
3. What are your impressions of the patient from the preliminary interview?

Case #2

Thomas Gabel, male, white, age 38, married

Diagnosis: unspecified neurological problem: suspect MS

Order: Patient causing problems on ward, uncooperative with nursing staff. Request recommendations regarding provision of recreation service. Patient has some manual limitations.

Notes: 6/14—Introduced by Dr. R. to Mr. Gabel during grand rounds. Gabel in semi-private room, but alone. Made appointment for interview on following day. Gabel grabbed my hand and would not let go while talking. Did not say more than a few words about being happy to talk with me. Dr. R. implied that it was mandatory that he make an appointment with me.

6/15—I did not extend my hand as I had done on the previous visit. Mr. G. made no attempt to grab at my hand, but grabbed my arm once during interview, to place emphasis on what he was saying. He appears to be rather intelligent in his conversation, well-read, etc., but quite angry about many things. His tone is hostile most of the time. He had just finished eating breakfast as I came in. I commented that he hadn't finished. He stated that there was no one to "serve him" so he couldn't finish. I said I would help him with his coffee cup. I showed him how he might drink his coffee by himself, if the cup were placed high enough on the bedside table and he sipped through a straw. He seemed pleased with this idea. He asked to have the pillows fixed and the bed lowered. I asked if there was anything else he wanted before we began to talk about activities. He then launched into a tirade about the problems he was having with nursing personnel. I repeated that I was not a nurse, and I was just helping him to be as comfortable as possible before we began our talk.

He then said he had one more request to make before we began our discussion. I asked him what that was. He asked if I were aware of the "one truth." I told him I didn't know what he meant. He began talking about Mary Baker Eddy and said that we were all sons of one father, and that he and I were brothers. I told him my father and his father were two different people, and I wasn't his brother. He got very angry at that and I pointed out that he was entitled to his opinion and I to mine. His anger dissipated, and he expressed some surprise. I asked him to tell me about himself. He replied, "You haven't given me enough time to prepare a lie!" I asked him what he meant by that. He asked me what I wanted to know. I asked about his work. He told me of his textile business and his responsibility in the business. His discussion was filled with sighs and pedantic phrases. I asked why he was so annoyed with me, since we hardly knew one another. He again looked surprised and began to smile. I said that if he had difficulty talking, we could stop. Throughout the rest of the discussion his speech softened and was less clipped, more fluid, a bit slurred in places, and he did not yell at me anymore.

We talked about his interests in literature and he asked me many questions. At one point he exclaimed with great surprise, "You seemed to have had an education!" We discussed his inability to hold a book and read, and about the talking book program. He wants to do this, and is going to think about which books he would like to " . . .read with his ears." I told him I'd see him in a couple of days, and we could talk about other things that might interest him, and that he might like to do.

Impression: Thinking seems clear and intact. He looks a mess—3-day growth of beard, hair uncombed, body covered with perspiration, bed sheets wet and disheveled, seems sufficient cause for irritation with personnel. His attitude also seems condescending toward staff. Ward personnel may be his intellectual inferior which may have a bearing on situation. He is severely rejected by staff (scuttlebutt picked up in nursing station); even though they do what they can for him, their attitude seems to transfer feelings of rejection and he responds with more demands and anger. I will try to give him a chance to use abilities that are dormant due to hospitalization, and try to create interest in activities that will use up some of the energy that is causing tension between him and ward staff.

6/20—Visited Mr. G. in the late afternoon. Brought the talking book machine and other equipment. He seemed glad to see me. Situation was rather bizarre. He was sitting in a chair holding onto his penis. A nurse standing by, quickly pulled his hand away and closed his pajamas. I ignored this and began to demonstrate the use of the equipment. The nurse then walked out of the room. As she did, he quickly began whispering that he wanted to see the head nurse, and that his nurse wouldn't let him. He said that nobody would let him see anyone anymore, that he was being held incommunicado, and could I please see if something could be done about this. He began to cry and seemed quite upset. I told him I would talk to Dr. R. about this and perhaps he could make some arrangements for him. I drew his attention to the equipment and asked if he had access to a set of earphones at home. He said he had a set of his own at home. I asked him to ask his wife to bring them. At this he became very upset, and screamed, "I can't do that, because I *love* her too much." He started to cry again. I couldn't get him to stop. I left the room and went to the nurse's station for assistance. In the station, the nurse said that this was a terribly difficult situation, and obviously all of the ward staff were alienated, and quite openly hostile to Mr. G. at this time. The nurse talked about the "poor" other patients and how difficult and impossible it was for them to tolerate this kind of thing.

Impression: Patient seems quite upset and overwrought, suspicious of everyone. No longer demanding, manifests childlike behavior and dependency. Where do we go from here?

6/22—Social Service note: Mr. T. Gabel, male, white, age 38, married. Patient converted Christian Scientist; severe neurological problems. Family does not believe in hospitals and have kept him away from medical care. Patient in advanced stage of multiple sclerosis. Discharged to private psychiatric hospital.

Questions

1. Is the physician's request appropriate?
2. Is the specialist really able to comply with this request?
3. What do you think of the specialist's way of talking with Mr. Gabel and responding to his outbursts?

CASE #3

Mary Jenns, female, white, age 99 and 4 mo., single

History: old hip fracture, recent ankle fracture; one cataract removed, one inoperable cataract; some hearing loss; curvature of the spine. Able to ambulate independently with a cane or a walker. Able to read regular print. Is extremely alert, with perfect recall of past and present. Compulsive talker, good sense of humor.

Recreation Summary Report: Miss J. is dismayed because she thought that "she was coming into a home, rather than a hospital." Finds the physical and mental state of others on her floor "depressing." Is somewhat distressed because she is having some difficulty getting to the bathroom "on time" late at night. (Nursing staff trying to help with this problem.) She reports that she deeply misses her nephew who lived with her, but is aware of the advantages of being in this "institution." Has been sewing on her own labels. Likes to go to the library, and indicates that she will attend other activities as soon as she becomes more familiar with her surroundings. She would like to get involved in discussion groups, and wonders if someone can show her where the different activities are held.

Attention Volunteer Department: Would it be possible to assign an escort to Miss J. for a few days, until she gets her bearings and learns her way around?

Questions

1. Should the recreation staff concern themselves with a person who is as old as Miss J. at the expense of younger patients?
2. Can someone this elderly really become involved in an ongoing discussion group?
3. What are some other activities that Miss J. might become involved in?

CASE #4

E. Hanks, female, white, age 77, married

Recreation Summary Report: July—Mrs. H. appears extremely weak, preoccupied, depressed, and says she wishes she could die. She is not interested in any of the activities but did say once that she likes to listen to recordings of Bach's music. She seems confused about the location of her room, and she claims that it doesn't make any difference whether anyone speaks to her or not; she "says" she doesn't hear them.

August—Mrs. H. stays in bed a good deal, and repeats that she is upset by the change in nursing personnel. Her son visited her during the month, but she indicated that this "isn't the same as a visit from a daughter." When asked why she stays in bed most of the time, she replied that she doesn't have much to wear. (This apparently is true—three pairs of her shoes have been stolen.)

September—Mrs. H. appears less depressed this month. She shared some poetry with other residents which her son had written to her. She has been using the portable phonograph to play some Bach. She prefers to stay in her room, but we are going to try to involve her in a more social atmosphere this month.

Questions

1. What responsibility does the recreation staff have for patients who prefer to engage in solitary activities within their own rooms?
2. Should the recreation staff attempt to "socialize" Mrs. H.?
3. Is it important whether a male recreation leader or female recreation leader be assigned to Mrs. H.? Explain your answer.

CASE #5

S. Ninkus, male, white, age 38, married

Diagnosis: undifferentiated psychosis

Order: Allow Mr. N. to become engaged in a number of recreation activities, report behavioral observations.

Recreation Progress Report: 3/17—Mr. N. is shy and introspective. Will stand in a room or sit without talking or will not participate in an activity unless direct reference is made to him. At times he will keep standing unless he is told to sit down. He appears to be constantly smiling. Although he seems intelligent enough, he does not show any initiative. He seems to focus his attentions upon the staff member who is directing an activity. He doesn't ask questions or volunteer information unless something is directed to him. He remains on the periphery of small groups. In a volleyball game when the ball is hit to him, he doesn't move until the ball is inches from him and then strikes out and hits the ball in a mechanical way. It is almost as if he is unaware the ball is coming until the last few seconds, or if he is aware, that he can't physically respond fast enough. He is involved in the group that is developing a newspaper, and he is like a machine in that he does not contribute to the conversation, but will take down what everyone has said if minutely directed to do this, or fold and staple reams of paper until told to stop. When he has been taken on trips out of the hospital, he exhibits the same type of behavior as in daily sessions in the hospital.

6/30—Mr. N. continues in same activities and also is helping to shelve books in the library. Staff noted increased spasmatic, uncontrolled, jerky movements of his body. Considerable amount of standing and staring. Later in the month these bodily movements decreased and are now absent. Speech was explosive, but has now become more fluid and he initiates conversations. He

Aspects of Professional Practice

seems to be more zestful, and moves into group discussions more easily. He no longer stands and stares at things or people. He seems to be a changed person.

9/20—Mr. N. again exhibiting involuntary muscular movements. He acts like a robot most of the time, with the current turned off! When someone speaks to him, his speech is normal and fluid as if the current has just been turned on. When he is asked to do something, he does it, but the instant the task is completed, it's like turning off the current again. He will stay in the last position he was in when he finished the task, and stares until further instructions are given. There seems to be nothing spontaneous about him whatsoever. There have been times when he has been left in a room by accident with the lights turned off, and on coming back a half hour later and turning on the lights, staff have found Mr. N. in the exact spot, not having moved an inch. He still continues to participate in many activities. He comes to dances and parties, and does not appear to be disturbed by his behavior. Others in the situation are very concerned and express this concern to staff. He is having more difficulty in establishing and maintaining social relationships each day. Apparently, his behavior is anxiety-provoking even to those who have known him for a few months. We note considerable rejection from fellow patients and volunteers.

Questions

1. What rationale might one give for the change in Mr. N.'s behavior during the month of June?
2. Should the recreation staff attempt to allay the fears of other patients regarding Mr. N.'s behavior, and if so, how can they do this?
3. In what ways are the recreation staff contributing to Mr. N.'s well-being?

CASE #6

Andy Richards, male, white, age 17 years 6 mo., height 5' 6", Weight 132 lbs., single

Diagnosis: mild mental retardation

General Appearance: Awkwardly thin and gangling, ill-clad, poorly groomed, facial acne, looks younger than his age, has a rather self-deprecating way of carrying himself and looking at you.

Social History: Lower middle-income laboring class, Scotch-Irish and Italian descent, Catholic family, youngest of three living children, fourth of five children born to the mother, history of being mother and sister's helper, easily distracted as a child, not meeting father's expectations, friend age 13, special education in public school. Father moved family to this city from a neighboring city to take position as a lithographer with a local printing firm. Father is a rather athletic man, interested in "keeping fit." Mother is a religious woman, sister is a nun, and a cousin is a priest. Mother is close to own family. Says Andy is "a little slower than his brother John, but is a good boy." Father tried to get Andy interested in activities at the C.Y.O., but Andy didn't take to these. Father wants him to join the Holy Name Society as a junior. Andy has gone to one meeting and has not gone back. Social relationships consist of 13-year-old friend, whom Andy helps with paper route. Sometimes (Andy reports) he and friend go downtown and watch people go back and forth. Andy goes to movies by himself, sometimes twice a day.

Educational History: Special education since the second grade. Sister Ellen tried to help him with reading, but was unsuccessful. He was eager to play games throughout school, but not too successful. Liked music and singing best. Made some friends with other children in elementary school, but unable to maintain relationships.

Employment History: Brother got Andy job as stockroom boy in drugstore chain, in which he worked. Was not there very long, fired for making too many mistakes. Worked as an elevator operator in a department store for a few months, but fired for similar reasons. Now working as a helper on a delivery truck for a wholesale notions firm.

Current Situation: A few months ago Andy went to the Teen Program at the Community Center. He didn't know anyone, so he didn't stay too long. He wanted to go to the dance they were having, but he didn't know how to dance. (Last year he thought if he knew how to dance he would be invited to some of the parties girls in his neighborhood were giving. He heard about the SS Dance School, and watched their commercials on TV. He went down to the studio and asked about dancing lessons. He couldn't read the contract he signed, but the next night he found out about its contents. It seemed that Andy had signed up for a $400 dance course, and the bill was sent to his father because he was a minor.) Thus, currently, dancing is somewhat of a traumatic notion in Andy's life.

He did have one date a couple of months ago. His mother arranged it with a girl in the neighborhood. Andy indicates that she was pleasant, but "talked too much." He had great difficulty in talking to her. He took her to the movies, but was quite nervous, and kept dropping candy and popcorn on her dress during the evening. He has tried to take her out again, but she tells Andy that she is very busy.

An uncle of Andy's who works in a bookbindery has told him about a better position there. He could arrange for Andy to join the union, and he has suggested that Andy could be on the company bowling team, as well as take advantage of other company-run recreation activities. Andy has not expressed much interest.

Aspects of Professional Practice 223

Questions

1. What effect has the family on Andy's social independence?
2. What problems do you see if Andy's current social pattern is not altered?
3. What kinds of assistance should be offered to Andy to help him progress toward social independence?

CASE #7

B. Valley, female, white, age 49, single

Diagnosis: depressive reaction; suspect symptomic of psychosis

Recreation Progress Report: Patient has been involved in recreation activities for a period of two months. Has difficulty in all activities. Cannot talk without whining and is constantly making excuses for herself. Picks up after everyone and feels responsible for everyone. During a party game when a counter was lost, she felt that the game could not go on unless the counter was found. She would not leave the room at the end of the party until the counter was found.

Unless asked to sit elsewhere, she chooses chairs on the edge of the room. She is neat and orderly about her looks, constantly brushing her hair with her hand. She says she is worried that she does nothing right and that she is making mistakes. She praises everyone and derides herself. She is unimaginative and behaves in a lethargic manner. Most of the time she is very cautious and reserved. She refuses to dance, be involved in dramatic activities, in fact she will enter into few activities. She constantly goes to the bathroom, but is only there a short time. Student nurses on duty report that she is usually washing her hands, but Miss R. has reported that patient masturbates in the bathroom.

Patient becomes upset when ashes are flicked on the floor by someone who is smoking, and she created a scene when coffee was accidentally spilled a few days ago, and had to be taken back to her room.

Request direction; recreation staff does not feel they are able to effect any change in this patient's behavior.

Questions

1. Which activities are particularly difficult for this patient to become engaged in? Explain your answer.
2. Why does the recreation staff feel they are unable to effect any change in behavior?

3. Should the recreation staff have behavioral change as an objective, or another objective?

CASE #8

R. Peratona, male, white, age 44, married

Background: Admitted to this hospital on 4/29 and placed on a medical service with a diagnosis of hypertension. Physician suggested that during the "work-up" period, he relax and take things easy. After some discussion, the physician told him that he might see if the recreation department could offer some suggestions for an hour of activity in the morning and two hours in the afternoon each day. The physician wrote such an order, and called the recreation department to specify that "The patient is rather an anxious person—see if you can get him to take it easy!"

Recreation Progress Notes: Mr. P. came to see the recreation specialist on 4/30. He appeared to be a man in his mid-forties, was rather stout, and pleasant to talk with. He talked a lot about how cooperative he had to be so that he could get well quickly and leave. He talked at great length about his interest in classical music. He explained that he knew a great deal about classical music and was very involved in music activities at the university. He was a language instructor at the university, but spent most of his time in the music department. It was decided that he would be able to use the music studio at the hospital and participate in a music listening program.

After a period of two weeks, it appeared that he didn't know as much about music as he said he did. He was constantly making excuses for his inadequacy. At this time an order was sent from his physician indicating that he was on a special diet, and he was not to eat anything when refreshments were served in the recreation department. Mr. P. understood this; however, it became apparent that he had to be carefully watched or he would "just have a few to see how they taste."

He complained a great deal to the recreation specialist about a patient in the next room to his, who finally died. Mr. P. said he did not sleep well because he had to lie awake listening to the patient moan. Now he has nightmares about this patient.

On 5/25, the recreation department received a notice that Mr. P. had been transferred from the medical service to the psychiatric service, and a request was made to furnish a summary report to Dr. M. On 6/27 the following report was sent by the recreation specialist:

In contact with other patients he assumes a rigid, autocratic, dictatorial role. He is verbose and difficult to shut up. In casual conversations with other

Aspects of Professional Practice

patients he goes to considerable lengths trying to prove his point of view, although this point of view is completely in the minority. After such a session he will tell the specialist that he is sorry this happened, but "the others are rather immature and have no understanding." He initiates considerable discussion about political problems. He assumes the role of "teacher of the world." He has the attitude that no one understands instructions as well as he, and so he must interpret the specialist's instructions to others during an activity. This occurs not only during small-group activity but in large mass activities as well. When limits are placed upon him, he responds with "Why must I?", but he respects the limits. His dress is becoming more bizarre. He now wears a necktie with his pajamas to evening activities. He complains incessantly about hospital routine. Most patients find him rather comical, and although they do not ridicule him to his face, express this behind his back. His discussions about women are filled with bravado. He tries to "teach" other male patients what women are "really" like, and where are the best places in the city to take them. He uses four-letter words spasmodically, but when other men patients initiate discussions regarding sexual experiences, he clams up.

Disposition: discharged to out-patient clinic on 7/20.

Note: Readmitted on 11/22; seems a lot quieter, more relaxed, passive.

Questions

1. How does Mr. P. relate to the recreation specialist? What role does he play with the specialist as compared with the other patients?
2. Is the original request for service regarding "relaxation" a reasonable request? Explain you answer.
3. What function can recreation service play in this situation now that Mr. P. has returned to the hospital?

CASE #9

Alice Thorton, female, white, age 19, height 5' 1", weight 106 lbs., single

Diagnosis: mental retardation (trainable)

General appearance: Attractive, dark curly hair, good complexion, delicately boned, slight figure; well-dressed, looks like typical university coed, facial expression marred by vacant appearance and constant inappropriate smile; sits with shoulders hunched and head turned away unless spoken to directly.

Social History: Upper middle-income professional family; father university professor, mother active clubwoman and socialite; obvious parental rejection; spent time in state institution; a private residential school, has been enrolled in Center program for two months. Mother finds it difficult to be Alice's mother in public and covers feelings of guilt with anger. Father overprotects Alice, full of self-pity and feelings of helplessness and hopelessness.

Probably fosters similar feelings in Alice, who acts more helpless and hopelessly inadequate than is warranted by her actual limitations.

Father reports that after Alice was born and they found out about her condition, considerable discord developed between him and his wife, and their marriage turned "sour." They sent Alice to the state school when she was age two and brought her home again when she was eight years old. He feels that this didn't help Alice, but helped them. "We could have done more for her, but we didn't, we did more for ourselves." After a year, they enrolled her in a private residential school because "it started all over again, the family, the neighbors. Everyone made life unbearable. The private school was the only answer." Father feels that the school was good for Alice, in that she looked better and seemed happier there. They brought her home at age sixteen. However, apparently this created new problems. "There was a horrible row when Alice began to scrub the kitchen floor. My wife kept trying to explain that that was the maid's job. I couldn't stand to see Alice sit there, day after day looking out of a window or twisting that piece of string. I told my wife that if all she could do was housework, let her do housework. We had a terrible battle. My wife would have none of it. After a few months, we agreed to allow Alice to come to the Sheltered Workshop program."

Current Situation: Alice has her own room, her own television set, good wardrobe, etc. Sheltered Workshop counselor reports that they could place her in a viable job, but parents refuse. Alice attends sheltered recreation program at the Center two nights a week. She is an active participant, plays games, sings, and dances. Parents won't allow her to join swimming parties. They will not permit her to go to the movies by herself and express fears that men will take advantage of Alice if they permit her to engage in unsheltered social situations.

Questions

1. What types of service have been missing in the state school and the private school that would have helped reduce or minimize Alice's social dependence?
2. What service should have been offered to Alice's family when she was younger to prevent some of the current problems, and what might be done today as a remedial effort?
3. Is it realistic of her parents to fear that men will take advantage of her, and what service might be offered to Alice to prevent this from happening?

CASE #10

Thomas Yorker, male, white, age 23, single

Diagnosis: possible psychosis

Aspects of Professional Practice

Order: Patient receiving diagnostic workup; is withdrawn, has problems relating to masculinity. Has been a university student. Evaluate for recreation service.

Recreation Report: 1/7—Specialist interviewed patient in his room on the ward. Patient was relaxing in bed, sitting upright in one corner. Bed was placed against wall, so patient was barely visible in the room without looking around corner of the door. Patient has private room. Nurse introduced specialist to patient. Patient sat up and shook hands; spoke in low tones; gave specialist fleeting glances throughout interview. Spoke hesitatingly with care and deliberation. Hair a bit unkempt, was in pajamas, paperback book lay on bed.

Commented about the patient's interest in reading, but got no response other than a shaking of the head. Asked about patient's major at the university. Patient stated that he went to school there and later worked in the offices; was studying psychology and switched to philosophy; finally dropped both because he "was inadequate to pursue a higher education any longer." He said he decided that he would have to find work since he "was getting too old to be a student." He took an office job to earn a living. Patient stated that he found it difficult to concentrate on his studies and went to a counselor. This didn't help—he still couldn't study and hoped the psychiatrist here could help him. Specialist commented that the patient found he had problems which kept him from studying. Patient then said he abandoned studies because "I found things in books which disturbed my thinking and conflicted with my ideas. I am not ready for this yet and I'll wait until later in life to change my ideas—until it is the proper time to make a decision." Asked when he knew it would be the right time to make a decision and what decision was he talking about. Patient answered that he would know, and wouldn't discuss this further. Patient lit a cigarette and moved around on the bed.

Asked about past educational experience. Patient said he went to parochial grammar and high school, did not participate in extracurricular activities, only academic subjects, and didn't do a good job of that. Asked patient if it bothered him that he did not participate in parties or athletics or other school activities. Patient said that it did, but that he was afraid to go since he did not know what would happen. Responded that activities bothered him. He said he made friends at the university but not in high school. He said he went to the rooms of his university friends and listened to records and talked about courses they were taking. He didn't go to parties, but found pleasure in visiting one or another of his classmates to study. Asked what else he did with these friends, patient would not respond.

Said that since patient was interested in music he might like to look at the collection of recordings in the music room. Patient did not appear to be particularly receptive or interested, but said he might do that. Mentioned some other activities that could be made available to the patient and invited him to come to the recreation department to discuss this at any time. Patient said thank you, got off the bed to shake hands, and said goodbye.

1/13—On recommendation of Dr. D., patient came to see specialist. He would like to have an opportunity to sit and listen to phonograph records. Scheduled use of small listening room one hour each afternoon. Patient requested that he be permitted to use equipment by himself. Specialist agreed.

1/23—Patient has been coming to listen to music each afternoon for almost two weeks. He is cordial but reserved. Does not discuss his personal problems. Sometimes another patient asks him if he may listen to a record with him. Patient agrees, but does not interact with the other patient. When three or four patients want to do this, he leaves the room and goes back to his room. He has discussed this with the specialist. He states in a very matter-of-fact way that he doesn't want to be with a number of other people. He says he cannot concentrate on more than one thing at a time and the talk of the others distracts him from the music. A volunteer has been assigned to begin to establish a relationship with him. The volunteer is a rather attractive, middle-aged woman. She offered him coffee three days in a row. Yesterday, he took it. Today he asked for her because she was late. She stayed with him about ten minutes and discussed some music and a book. She will try to lengthen the time tomorrow. We plan to get him to tolerate her for at least an hour, and share the activity with her. We will try to move others into the session and get the patient involved in other activities by the end of the month.

Questions

1. How "sick" is this patient?
2. Was the specialist's probing during the initial interview appropriate?
3. What theoretical rationale can you find for the method being employed as described in the material on 1/23?

CASE #11

F. Hendel, female, white, age 71, married

Diagnosis: hip fracture

Order: Patient will be in a body brace for an undetermined period. Try and get her interested in a variety of activities to keep her mind off her brace. She is an alert and intelligent woman.

Recreation Report: During July Mrs. H. was interested in being taken out of her room to the garden, but "not by those ten-year-olds" (our teen volunteers who are part of the community cooperation unit). In discussion with

Aspects of Professional Practice   229

the recreation specialist she was pleasant and articulate. She complained about never having had the experience of being around Negroes before coming to the Home, and said that she finds the encounter unpleasant. She said that she would rather be completely without her senses than to be in her present state. She feels that she is not as bright as she has been. She expresses concern about the condition of other residents on her floor. She indicated that she would like to do some "handcrafts," but she says she is unable to use her hands.

Since August, Mrs. H. has become increasingly preoccupied by the discomfort caused by her supportive girdle-brace and has come to feel that the lack of attention given by staff in obtaining a new brace for her is evidence of her "hopeless situation."

In early September, she was evaluated by the physiatrist, Dr. S., and it was decided that a new brace should be made for her. In conversations with the recreation specialist, she keeps insisting that nothing will be done, and that she will not be given a new brace. Lately, she has frequently been seen without her dentures. She no longer is concerned with her appearance, and seems to have lost her composure and dignity. We have tried on several occasions to engage her in a number of activities, but she continues to resist.

We would appreciate an evaluation of her mental state and would like to know if she is receiving medication that has caused the behavioral decline. Shall we continue to take the approach with her that we have been using, or should we alter our approach?

Questions

1. Is it appropriate for the recreation staff to request an evaluation of the patient's mental state and ask about the medication she is receiving? Explain your answer.
2. How would you respond to her comments about the volunteers?
3. If the physician indicates that another approach should be taken, what approach would you use?

CASE #12

Thomas Faftner, male, white, age 28, married, 2 children

Diagnosis: quadriplegic (post-polio)

Order: Patient will be receiving medical evaluation and subsequently full range of rehabilitation services. It is not clear at this time how much functional gain can be expected. Establish a relationship with the patient and determine types of activities he engaged in, and which may be possible for future involvement.

Report of Preliminary Recreation Interview: Met with patient at 6:15 P.M. Patient appeared bright and cheery and returned my greeting. He was lying in bed listening to the radio. After introducing myself, I asked him to tell me about himself. He said he was a college graduate from the University of Southhampton, that he was married and had two very young children. He said while he was in high school he participated in athletics and in a number of music groups. He played the pipe organ, the accordion, and the piano. He met his wife while he was in University, and married her when they were in attendance. He said that his wife and children are staying in a motel while he is here in the hospital. He said he was very concerned about finding them a place to live close by since he would be here quite a while. He said he wanted them to be close to him, but how could he help them now. He felt that his savings were dwindling fast. I asked him if he had talked to anyone in social service about this. He said he had. He asked if I knew of any cheap apartments nearby which they could rent, and could I help him with this. I replied that I wasn't qualified to help him with this problem, but that social service was, and I was sure they would do this for him. He seemed rather anxious. I changed the subject by asking him about his reading habits, since I noticed a book by the side of his bed. He said that his wife was reading the *Silver Chalice* to him when she came to see him each evening after the children were asleep. He said that he supposed lying in bed gave him a "golden opportunity" to catch up on his reading, if only he could hold a book. I talked about the number of devices we had for assisting with reading, and discussed the Hundred Great Books program. He said that he knew so little, and that sounded like something he'd like to do. I said I would get some more information to him about the program. He said he would appreciate it since the time went so slowly in the hospital. He said he liked to read the newspapers, but couldn't hold them. He then volunteered that he was also interested in photography and had quite a collection of colored slides which he had taken in Europe. He said he thought that it might be fun to see some slides that others had taken of places he has been. He then said Europe was the place he got sick. He explained that he was working there, and it happened without any warning. He said he supposed that he could never go back to his job again, or do most of the things he used to do. He said he was really getting some first-hand experience of how a hospital was run, and perhaps he could get a job in a hospital when he was no longer a patient. He thanked me for visiting him, and said he would look forward to seeing me again.

Questions

1. In your opinion, how well do you think the specialist handled the issue of the apartment? Should he have allowed the patient to talk about this at length?
2. Are the activities in which the patient engaged in the past possible for future involvement?

Aspects of Professional Practice

3. What type of activity program would you recommend for this patient?

CASE #13

Arnold Mack, male, Negro, age 40, single

Diagnosis: receiving work-up for unspecified emotional complaints; manifests some GI disturbance

Social History: Patient works as superintendent in an office building. Lives alone.

Recreation Report: (Patient has been involved in a variety of activity sessions over the past month. The following is an extract for one day.)

Patient came to the specialist's office and asked him if he would do him a favor. The specialist said that depended on what it was. The patient asked if the specialist would go to the OT shop and get his lamp so that he could take it to his room and finish it. The shade was being made in OT and the rest of the lamp was being made in the craft shop on his ward. Specialist asked him why he didn't go himself. Patient replied that he was afraid to. Specialist said he wouldn't go. Patient asked if the specialist would go with him. Specialist said no, and asked what was bothering him—why was he afraid to go to OT. Patient said that he was fine when it came to recreation service or working in the craft shop, but he did not know what was wrong about OT. Specialist asked if he discussed this with his doctor, and he replied that he did, but the doctor didn't understand it either. He said he seemed to get along fine with the men on the staff, but not with the women. When asked if this included the nursing staff, he said that was different. He said he didn't want people to think he was "strange." He said that people usually thought he was "ugly," but that "there is a power in ugliness." Specialist asked if he felt the OT's didn't like him. He looked up and said, "One has to be careful of what one says." Specialist reassured him that it was alright to speak freely, and say how he felt. The patient said, "I have to be careful of offending white women." Specialist asked if he told this to his doctor. Patient said no. Specialist asked why. Patient looked surprised and replied "My doctor is a white woman." The specialist said that the doctor was here to help him and should not be thought of as a woman, only as his doctor. Patient replied, "The ladies in OT are here to help also." Specialist asked if he thought that the ladies in OT didn't like him because he was a black. He replied that he didn't know, but if he accidentally touched them, they pulled away rapidly. Patient said now that this was out, he was glad. He then talked a good bit about how it felt to be in the minority, and how the OT's made him feel. Specialist suggested that he talk with the doctor about this. Patient said he couldn't. Specialist said that he would tell the doctor about this conversation. Patient asked him not to. Specialist said that he would rather the patient discussed it with the doctor, and he would wait at least two days to say anything. Specialist then asked couldn't patient go and get his lamp now? Patient said he thought he could. He said thank you and left.

Questions

1. Should the specialist have allowed the patient to discuss these things with him? Explain your answer.
2. Should the specialist have gone with him to get his lamp? Why?
3. Should the specialist tell the doctor about this conversation?

CASE #14

Fredrick Sturbridge, male, white, age 17, single

Diagnosis: cerebral palsy

General Appearance and Condition: Obese, multiple disability which has affected ambulation and intelligence; uses wheelchair; well-dressed, obvious dental caries, poor general hygiene, some visual problems.

Social History: Middle-income family, special education in public school when family can arrange it. Parents are in their 50s; child is dependent in all areas; mother is impatient; father concentrates on his work, doesn't spend much time with the boy; child is and will be vocationally and socially dependent; spends considerable time by himself with nothing to do, no friends; parents lack knowledge and imagination, and are at a loss.

Educational History: It is difficult to determine how retarded Freddy is. He has learned to read on approximately a third-grade level and should enjoy newspaper pictures and headlines. He may be able to read content such as is found on the sports page. He has been taught to take certain responsibilities in the home.

Recreation Report: Because he has no friends and his parents take little interest in him, he spends almost all day watching television, or the people who go by his window. (He lives in a first-floor flat.) Parents say he has been taught to use crutches but he doesn't practice with them, and they find it too much trouble to insist since "he is in that condition." He has gone on vacation to his grandfather's farm each summer, but he says it's just like being at home only he spends some time outside. His father tried to take him out a few times to watch some sporting events, but there was some difficulty about the fire laws and the wheelchair. When asked about such things as a windowbox garden, or swimming, or a camp for disabled children, his mother said they all seem like things that might interest Freddy, but she or his father wouldn't know where to begin.

Questions

1. Do you feel that Freddy should remain at home or be institutionalized? Explain your answer.

Aspects of Professional Practice

2. What makes Freddy as dependent as he is?
3. If you were assigned to this case, what would you do in the event that Freddy must remain at home?

CASE #15

Charles Morris, male, Negro, age 25, single

Diagnosis: unspecified GI disturbance

Order: Patient has an emotional problem, but cannot talk about it. Place in a variety of recreation activities so that he has realistic material for use in psychotherapy sessions.

Recreation Report: Mr. Morris is an extremely polite and industrious person. He has become a member of a music listening group, among other activities. He is most interested in assisting in cataloging phonograph records. He expresses a good degree of individual creativeness and ability. After his natural anxiety abated in regard to the group, he began taking an active part. It is interesting to note that before he became involved with this group, he did not possess any prior knowledge of classical music. He now receives considerable praise from other patients and staff. He is becoming somewhat of an expert on Mozart. He functions superficially in intragroup relations however, responding only to assignments. There is still somewhat of a strain on a verbal level. He will enter into discussions, and will start out impartially, but eventually will side with whatever point of view the recreation specialist advocates. He keeps remarking about how amazed he is with some of the things that seem to come up for casual discussion. When the patients initiate something that has a sexual content, Mr. Morris listens but won't get involved in the discussion. He refuses to get angry with anyone, though at times he has had ample cause. The recreation specialist has attempted to generate anger, but he does not respond. He constantly tells the specialist that he "has a great deal to learn" and he appreciates the chance being offered to him. He expresses enthusiasm about dances, parties, entertainments, lectures, and other special events in the program. He is a passive spectator at all of these events, not an active participant. When he comes to an activity after a psychotherapy hour, his behavior is no different than before. He tells others "how grand the doctor is," "how good it is to talk over problems with someone," and "everyone should have this opportunity."

Questions

1. Is the physician's request for service a realistic one?
2. Should the specialist try to intentionally anger Mr. Morris for this purpose?
3. What other techniques might the specialist employ with respect to this request?

Index of Names

Ackoff, R., 128
Acuff, S.H., 96
Adams, R.C., 212
Adatto, C., 212
Aesclepiades of Bithynia, 6
Aesculapius, 5
Albee, G.W., 10
Archer, J., 212
Arje, F.B., 2, 96, 209
Armstrong, R.J., 154
Aschrott, P.F., 9
Avedon, E.M., 2, 23, 62, 74, 209
Avicenna, 8

Baldwin, A.L., 112
Bales, R.F., 172
Banathy, B., 129, 134, 135, 139
Barclay, D., 212
Bauer, D., 212
Beisser, A., 212
Beresford, A., 212
Bergler, E., 212
Bevans, J.E., 212
Biddle, W.W., 62
Bieren, J., 97
Blau, L., 212
Boeshart, L.K., 212

Boggs, E., 18
Borgatta, E.F., 172
Boyd, N., 14, 212
Braaten, J., 212
Brachman, D.S., 212
Brightbill, C.K., 106
Brown, M.E., 212
Brown, R.L., 212
Browne, W.A.F., 5, 10
Buell, C.E., 213

Calvin, J., 44
Campbell, R.J., 24
Carlson, G., 213
Carlson, R.E., 106
Carr, A.C., 213
Carroccio, D.F., 213
Cartwright, D., 172
Case, M., 13
Cervantes, 1
Chapman, F.M., 213
Charaka, 8
Chiron, 5
Colb, K.M., 213

Dahl, G.J., 44
Danford, H.G., 106

Index of Names

Daniel, A., 212
Daniel, G., 22
Danning, E., 213
David, 2
De Schweinitz, K., 83
De Schweintz, E., 83
Delany, E., 213
Demarche, D.F., 62
Deppe, T.R., 106
Dewey, J., 202
Dichter, E., 120, 121
Dominick, J.R., 78
Don Quixote, 1

Eckman, D.P., 133
Esquirol, 10
Evans, K.E., 103

Feigenbaum, K., 115
Fell, J.H., 213
Fleixson, R.S., 97
Fox, S.S., 213
Frankel, G., 213
Frankel, L. 213
Freud, S., 203
Fromm, E., 25, 203
Frye, V., 106

Gagne, R.M., 154
Galen, 6,9
Gardner, G.E., 110
Garrett, W.A., 115
Garrison, M., 201
Ginglend, D., 213
Goffman, E., 119, 120, 121
Goldsmith, S., 72
Goshen, C.E., 119
Gray, P.E., 213
Greenblatt, M., 98
Gronlund, N.E., 154
Guilford, J.P., 200, 201, 202, 203
Gump, P.V., 213
Gunzberg, 203
Guthrie, D., 8
Guttman, L. 14

Hamlet, 171
Hare, A.P., 172
Haun, Paul, 1, 2, 15, 19, 20, 209
Havinghurst, R.J., 115
Hill, B.H., 15, 18
Hitch, C.J., 154

Hoepfner, R., 200, 201
Homachea, C.R., 16
Hopeman, R., 128
Hua T'o, 6, 7, 8
Hume, E.H., 8
Hyde, R.W., 213

Johns, R., 62
Jokl, E., 213
Jung, C.G., 203

Kaegi, A., 8
Kazanjian, S.S., 70
Keffer, L., 213
Kelley, H.H., 172
Kessing, F.M., 45, 49
Kirkbride, T., 118, 119
Klinger, J.L., 73
Knight, J.A., 214
Knowles, H., 172
Knowles, M., 172
Kramer, B.M., 98
Kraus, R.G., 44, 49, 106
Kubie, S.H., 15

Lamonte, J.L., 9
Landau, G., 15
Landy, D., 98
Langdon, G., 89
Lee, I., 212
Leland, H., 202
Levinson, T., 78
Lindner, S., 45
Lindsay, Z., 213
Lowman, E., 73
Luther, M., 44

MacLean, J.R., 106
Mager, R.F., 154
Martin, A.R., 15, 24, 48
Martin, F.W., 75
McBain, R.L., 212
McCormack, J.B., 57
McCormic, J.B., 96
McKindree, O.J., 214
McMullin, M.D., 101
Mead, M., 113
Melampus, 5
Menninger, W., 24
Meyer, H., 15
Meyer, H.D., 106
Meyer, M.W., 18

Index of Names

Mignoga, M., 214
Miles, M.B., 172
Milita, E.J., 214
Miller, I., 101, 176

Nightingale, F., 13

O'Morrow, G.S., 57, 96
Olsen, W.E., 57
Olsen, W.L., 96

Palmer, M., 96
Parker, D., 214
Parker, S., 45
Pepys, Samuel, 22
Peters, M., 106
Peterson, C.A., 128
Piaget, J., 202
Pinel, P., 10
Plant, J., 24, 48
Plato, 6
Pomeroy, J., 106
Proteus, 5
Pythagoras, 6
Pytherch, H., 214

Quade, E.S., 136
Quattlebaum, L.F., 213

Raymond, E.B., 214
Rensvold, V., 18
Rich, M.K., 101
Richardson, U., 214
Roberts, K., 49
Robinson, R., 62
Roderman, C.R., 214
Rodney, L.S., 106
Roger, G., 214
Rogers, C., 203
Rullman, L., 212
Rusalem, H., 73
Rusk, H.A., 16
Ryland, G., 111

San Kuo Chih, 6, 7
Sanders, I., 62
Sapora, A.W., 214

Saul, 2
Schattner, R., 214
Schlotter, B., 14
Schwartz, A., 101
Scott, M.G., 177
Sereny, G., 78
Shakespeare, 2
Sieder, V.M., 62
Slovenko, R., 214
Smith, R.G., 154
Soranus, 6
Spiers, 203
Stafford, G.T., 214
Stiles, W.E., 213
Stock, D., 172
Stone, W.C., 214
Stotsky, B.A., 78
Sullivan, H.S., 203
Summers, L., 13
Sutton-Smith, B., 23, 213

Thelen, H.A., 172
Thibaut, J.W., 172
Thomas, G., 214
Tilgher, A., 44
Tyler, R.W., 155

Verstrate, D., 176

Wallace, S.E., 120
Warren, R.L., 62
Webb, B., 9
Webb, S., 9
Weber, M., 44
Weinberg, W.L., 70
Wells, W.D., 115
Wickwire, G.C., 182
Wilson, G., 111
Wisher, P.R., 214
Wolf, G., 214
Wolffe, J., 15
Wood, A., 214
Woodward, H.H., 214
Wrightson, H.A., 13, 214

Yueng-hung, M., 213

Zander, A., 172

Index of Titles

Anatomist, 200
Anthropologist, 23

Beggar, 22

Consultant, 66, 67, 68, 69, 70, 71, 150
Correctionalist, 76, 81
Criminologist, 81

Dietician, 108

Educator, 32, 76, 81
   adult, 33
   homestudy, 87
   outdoor, 34
   physical, 19, 34
      adaptive, 34
      corrective, 34
   special, 19, 33
   teacher, 67

Folklorist, 23

Gypsies, 21

Housekeeper, 57

Idlers, able bodied, 21

Interpreter, 85

Librarian, 9

Mathematician, ancient, 6

Ne'Er do wells, 21
Nurse, 20, 61, 67, 76, 77, 81, 85, 93, 96, 99, 108, 120, 122, 150
   student, 75

Parents, nondisabled children, 73
Parolees, 98
Personnel, subprofessional, 75
Physician, 67, 81, 85, 86, 92, 95, 202, 204
   Ancient:
      Chinese, 6
      Greek, 6
      Indian, 8
      Persian, 8
   French, 10
   intern, 75
   internist, 87
   legendary, 5
   physiatrist, 16, 19
   psychiatrist, 48, 207
   writer, 16

Index of Titles

Playground, supervisor, 73
Poet, 1
Priest, 92
Program director, 108, 109
Psychoanalist, 203
Psychologist, 57, 77, 96, 200, 202, 207

Radiologist, 20
Rehabilitation counselor, 81, 96, 108, 198
Rehabilitationist, 76, 77

Servant, 2
Social work, 19, 35, 56, 59, 67, 76, 81, 83, 84, 91, 92, 93, 95, 96, 122, 150
  case work, 35, 108
  community organization, 36
  group work, 19, 35, 36
Sociologist, 48, 49
Speakers, 9
Storytellers, 9

Therapist:
  activity, 38
  art, 38
  corrective, 19, 38
  dance, 38
  drama, 38
  group-psycho, 78
  music, 38
  occupational, 19, 38, 78, 182
  physical, 19, 20, 38, 87, 108, 122, 123, 182
  play, 38
  psycho-, 123
  speech, 19
Tourist, 114
Treasurer, 22

Vagabonds, 21
Veteran, disabled, 14
Volunteer, 59, 75, 78, 97, 99, 100, 125, 126, 204, 205, 206
  groups, 108

Index of Places and Organizations

America, middle, 4
Ancient:
   Babylon, 4
   China, 6, 8
   Egypt, 5
      Nile River, 5
   Greece, 5, 6
   India, 6, 8
   Jericho, 4
   Lagash, 4
   Nineveh, 4
   Rome, 5, 6
      Bithynia, 6
   Ur, 4
Australia, organization,
   Parkland Hospital, 17

Canada, 2, 16, 17, 47, 53, 58, 126
   Alberta, 17
      Calgary, 17
      Edmonton, 17
   Ontario, 1, 78
   Quebec:
      Montreal, organization, recreation for the handicapped, 17
China, ancient, 6, 8
Crimea, 13

Denmark 53, 73

Egypt:
   ancient, 5
   Cairo, 8
   organization, Mansur Hospital, 8
England, 6, 9, 14, 17, 21, 44, 47, 58, 73, 203
   London Times, 3
   organization:
      Disabled Living Foundation, 73
      Spastic Society, 17
      Stoke Manderville, 14
   poor laws, 9, 22
Europe, 6, 8, 9, 10, 16, 17, 23
   Continental, 47
   Western, 2

Fertile Crescent, 5
Finland, 17
France, 9, 10, 58

Germany, 9, 58, 113
Greece, 113, 123
   ancient, 5
      Epidaurus, 5
Guatamala, 84

Index of Places and Organizations

India, 17
    Ancient, 6, 8
International organization:
    Red Cross, 13
Israel, 17
Italy, 58, 91

Japan, organization, 7, 17, 47
    Tokyo Suyama Hospital, 17

Kashmir, 8

Mexico, organization, 16
    Mexico City Hospital Infantil, 17
Middle East:
    Arab, 9
Moslem, 8

Netherlands, organization, 17, 53, 74, 203
    J. Henry Dunant Vacation Ship, 17
North America, 119
Norway, 123

Persia, 8
Phillippines, 17

Rome, ancient, 5, 6

Scotland:
    Glasgow organization, 10
        Gartnavel Royal Lunatic Asylum, 10
Spain, 1, 17, 85, 123
Sweden, 1, 17, 47, 73
    Stockholm, 17
Switzerland, 58

United States, 15, 47, 49, 53, 57, 58, 75, 77
    Nevada, 16
    New Jersey, 12
    New York City, 13, 15
    New York Times, 16
    organization:
        American Asso. on Mental Deficiency, 202

Organization, *cont.*
    American College of Sports Medicine, 15
    American Heart Association, 198
    American Psychiatric Asso. Comm. on Leisure, 15
    American Recreation Society, 75
    American Red Cross, 13
    Catholic Youth Organization, 87
    Comeback, Inc. 16, 76
    Federation of Women's Clubs, 207
    Goldwater Memorial Hospital, 15
    Industrial Home for the Blind, 13
    Jewish Guild for the Blind, 13
    Joseph Bulova School of Watchmaking, 15
    Junior Chamber of Commerce, 207
    Junior League, 207
    Minneapolis.
        Circle F Club, 98
    National Association of Recreation Therapists, 76
    National Recreation and Park Association, 76
    National Recreation Association, 15
    National Therapeutic Recreation Society, 76
    New York:
        City Department of Welfare, 15
        Fountain House, 98
        University, 14
    New York Association for the Blind, 13
    Philadelphia:
        Horizon House, 98
        Pennsylvania Hospital, 118
    Rotary International, 207
    San Francisco:
        Fellowship Club, 98
    Texas State Penitentiary, 16
    University of North Carolina, 15
    Veteran's Administration, 78
    Young Women's Christian Asso., 98

Western Hemisphere, 10

Index of Settings

Agency:
  aftercare, 98
  community, 18, 24, 63, 97, 100
    nonresidential, 122
    residential, 98
  coordinating, 67
  health, 100
    federation of, 62
  multigenerational service, 15
  multiservice, 64
  municipal, 64
  neighborhood, 18
  nonresidential, 100
  recreation, 50
    public/private, 17
  regional, 67
  rehabilitation, 98
    vocational, 81
  social, 97, 100
  social work, 36
Aquarium, 47
Arenas, 31, 47, 99

Beach, 47, 103
Bowling Alleys, 31
Building:
  county office, 31
  nonelevator, 101

Campsite, 31, 34, 103
Center:
  community, 15, 30, 33, 47
    mentally retarded, 61
    older adults, 15
    recreation, 58
  continued treatment, 93
  drop-in, 17
  mental health, 27
  recreation:
    for the blind, 13
    neighborhood, 102
  rehabilitation, 98
  senior, 31, 82, 88
  young adult, 61
Church, 30, 31, 33, 87, 88
  parish, 47
  Sunday school, 36
Circus, 31
Clinic, 16, 25, 34, 38
  outpatient, 38, 58
Club:
  country, 47
  golden age, 88
  private, 87
Convents, 2
Cooperative:
  farm, 50

Index of Settings

Department:
  health, 18, 50, 67
  recreation, 54, 55, 67
    municipal, 57, 62, 98
    public, 50, 59, 100
Dining room
  staff, 122

Facilities, recreation:
  community, 121
Family, 121

Golf course:
  public/private, 84
Guild:
  for the blind, 13

Halls:
  concert, 103
Hallway:
  deadend, 122
Homebound:
  program for the, 16
Houses:
  halfway, 98
Housing project, 88

Institutions (*see also* Schools), 108
  asylum, 10
  for the blind, 13, 14, 31
  congregate living, 117
  continuing care, 78
  correctional, 2, 16, 26, 27, 31, 50, 81, 84, 93, 98, 110
  for the deaf, 14
  educational, 52
  expressive, 27
  health, 52
  homes:
    for the aging, 27, 56, 112
    nursing, 16, 18, 31, 38, 63, 81, 84, 93
  hospital, 2, 8, 15, 18, 27, 31, 34, 38, 59, 87, 89, 90 110, 119, 120, 132
    clinic:
      homecare, 88
      outpatient, 86
    day, 98
    general, 57, 61, 89, 91
    military, 13, 14
    night, 98

Institutions, hospital, *cont.*
    psychiatric, 38, 57, 84, 89, 96, 99
    rehabilitation unit, 94
    veterans, 14
    ward, 13, 85
    weekend, 98
  instrumental, 27
  for the mentally ill, 13, 14
  for the mentally retarded, 12, 13, 14, 26, 31
  rehabilitation, 31
  residential, 2, 25, 26, 31, 34
    for the aging, 16
    long-term, 24, 52, 81, 93
    special, 18
  sanitoria, 2
  sanitorium:
    tuberculosis, 15
  task-oriented, 27, 52
  youth, 16

Lakes, 31
Landmarks:
  community, 117
Libraries, 47
Lighthouse, 13
Lot:
  parking, 122

Military bases, 30
Monasteries, 2
Mountains, 31
Museum, 47, 103

Parks, 30, 47, 58
  amusement, 31
  national, 34
  regional, 31, 34
Penitentiary (*see* Institutions, correctional)
Playground, 30, 72, 81
Pools, 47, 103, 175
Prison (*see* Institutions, correctional)
Program:
  agricultural-extension, 50
  for the noninstitutionalized, 16
  nonsheltered, 26
  rehabilitation, 14
  sheltered, 26
  transitional:
    social, 97
    urban, 50
Pubs, 31

Resorts, 31
Resources:
    commercial, 30
    home, 83
    neighborhood, 83
Restaurants, 31, 84, 103, 123
Rodeos, 31

Schools (see also Institutions), 30, 33, 50
    for the blind, 84, 93
    boarding, 34
    colleges, 34
        community, 53
    deaf, 82
    mentally retarded, 81, 93
    public, 34
    residential, 33
    rural, 31
    ships, 34
    special, 2, 18, 31
    state, 61
    technical institutes, 53
    training, 16
    universities, 53

Scouts, 47
Seashore, 31
Sheltered workshop, 16
Ships:
    school, 34
    vacation, 17
Shop:
    craft, 175
Snow areas, 31
Stadia, 31, 47
Store, department, 126
Synagogues, 30

Taverns, 31

Woodland areas, 31, 34
Work-place, 119
Workhouses, 9
Workshop, 25

Y's, 30, 47

Zoos, 47, 103

Index of Activities

Activity, 213
   art, 17, 73, 84, 164, 204, 205, 213, 214
      drawing, 184, 185, 190
      flower arranging, 118
      painting, 191
   coed, 16
   community service, 101
   cultural, 16
   family, 115
   play, 213
   social, 16, 17, 212
   winter, 122

Bench sitting, 58
Boating:
   canoeing, 187, 189, 193
   rowing, 187, 188, 189, 190, 192, 195, 197
Body-building, 210

Camping, 84, 212, 232
Clubs, 56
Cooking, 56
Crafts, 82, 88, 164, 165, 175, 204, 205
   basketry, 187
   bookbinding, 186
   carving, 184, 185, 186
   ceramics, 189, 190, 194

Crafts, *cont.*
   construction, 211
   construction set, 85
   crocheting, 184
   hammering, 183
   jewelry making, 183, 184, 186, 187
   knitting, 174
   leather work, 183, 184, 186, 187, 188
   pottery, 183, 184, 185, 186, 187, 188, 189, 194, 195, 196, 197, 198
   weaving, 174, 184, 185, 186, 187, 188, 189, 190, 191, 194, 195, 196, 197, 198
      basket, 183
      card, 183, 184
      loom, 183
   woodworking, 59, 183, 184, 185, 186, 187, 188, 189, 190, 191, 194, 196, 216, 231

Dancing, 4, 5, 6, 11, 16, 51, 61, 85, 96, 122, 175, 192, 193, 194, 196, 197, 206, 207, 214, 221, 226, 233
   balls, 10
   lessons, 222
   prohibitions, 9
   square, 186, 214

Dancing, *cont.*
  ward, 213
Daydreaming, 163
Dining out (*see also* Excursions), 45, 58, 84, 99, 162
Discussion groups, 56, 93, 219, 225
  great books, 58
Driving:
  sightseeing, 117

Entertain, 4, 45
Entertainers, 4
Entertainment, 233
Equipment:
  camera, 83, 87
  punching bag, 85
  tape recorder, 83
  television set, 87
Excursions (*see also* Theater), 5
  holiday cruise, 17
  meetings, 59
  restaurants, (*see also* Dining out), 56
  seaside, 17
  sight seeing, 17
  theater, 56
  traveling, 45
  vacations:
    country, 59

Fencing, 187, 188, 190, 192, 193, 194, 195, 196
Festivals, 4
  fairs, 9
Fishing, 187, 189, 192
  fly casting, 186

Games (*see also* Sports): 204, 205, 212, 214, 226
  active, 213
  bedside, 14, 212
  board, 4, 5, 210
    backgammon, 8
    checkers, 73, 166, 183, 185
    chess, 8, 87, 166, 206, 213
    go, 7
    parchisi, 8
    Wei-chi, 7
  box hockey, 87
  cat's cradle, 184
  children, 213
    "It", 167
    Jacks, 183, 193

Games, Children, *cont.*
  London Bridge, 23
  competitive, 74
  courtship, 23
  darts, 183, 184, 185, 192, 193
  education, 12
  equipment:
    cardholder, 73
  gambling, 4, 22, 51, 212
    bingo, 165
    cards, 9, 10, 59, 183, 184, 186, 187, 189, 204
      Blackjack, 206
      Bridge, 73, 170, 174, 175, 214
      Pinochle, 94, 95, 96
      Poker, 55, 82, 112, 168, 174
      Schafkopf, 113
    Casinos, 16, 123
    Chance, 9, 10
    Chicken, 209
    Dice, 8, 9
    Handycapp, 22
    Russian Roulette, 209
  Hitting, 85
  Hop Scotch, 194, 195
  Hospital, 14, 212
  House, 14
  Isthmian, 6
  Kicking, 85
  Motion, 212
  Muscle-Building, 213
  Olympic, 6
  party, 223
  puzzles, 206
    crossword, 210
    jigsaw, 5
    picture, 86
  relaxation, 6
  remedial, 212
  Ring Toss, 183, 184, 185, 188, 191
  running, 5
  shuffleboard, 87, 174, 183, 184, 188, 189, 190, 191, 192, 193
  skipping rope, 188, 197
  sound, 214
  table, 4, 5, 73
    dominoes, 10
    pool, 51
    tennis, 86
      ping pong, 184, 186, 187, 188, 194, 195, 206
  team, 175, 212

Index of Activities

Gardening, 5, 8, 73, 183, 184, 187, 190, 192, 193, 194, 195, 196, 197
   windowbox, 232
Grooming, 60, 61

Hiking, 196
Hobby, 117, 210
   shop, 95
   stamp collecting, 36, 83
Homework:
   helping with, 59

Inactivity, 120

Juggling, 4
Jumping, 197

Knitting, 88, 183, 210

Lecturers, 8
Lectures, 233
Library, 5
Loving, 45

Magic, 45
Marbles, 183
Movies, 16, 55, 87, 118, 165, 226
Music, 4, 6, 8, 9, 122, 212, 213
   band, 169
   bouzouki, 113
   choir, 169
   choral group, 102
   classical, 233
   concerts, 5, 10, 13, 56, 58, 59, 84, 103, 117
   equipment:
      harp, 2
      phonograph, 58
   listening to, 85, 91, 93, 204, 211
   orchestra, 17, 50
   phonograph:
      listening to, 206, 220, 227, 228
   piano playing, 91, 183, 185, 197, 207
   playing, 211
   religious, 216
   sing:
      community, 175
   singing, 226
   song, 4, 11
   strings, 183, 186
   theater, 17
   violin playing, 191, 192

Painting, 59
Parties, 55, 84, 122, 205, 207, 221, 233
Pets, 13
Photography, 92, 230
Picnics, 16
Play, 14
Playground:
   rooftop, 17
Playing, 45
Playrooms, 9
Playthings, 9
Poetry, 6

Radio, 17, 58
Radios, listening to, 88
Reading, 58, 88, 92, 115, 164, 183, 184, 186, 222, 230
   books, 9
      largeprint, 73
      talking, 58, 216, 218
   newspapers, 55
Reciting, 9
Reminiscing, 58
Resting, 45
   napping, 55
Riding:
   bicycle, 192, 194, 196, 197
   horseback, 195, 196, 211

Sewing, 184, 219
   embroidery, 183
   needlework 185
Shopping, 59, 60
Skating, 194
   ice, 196, 197
   roller, 195, 197
Spectator activities, 6
Sports (*see also* Games), 4, 16, 17, 22, 212, 213
   archery, 1, 178, 187, 189, 190, 191, 192
   athletics, 34, 38, 212
   badminton, 185, 189, 191
   ball, 59, 214
      court, 4
   ball games, 185, 186, 192, 193, 194 195, 197
   baseball, 187, 188, 189, 190, 191, 192, 194, 196, 197
   basketball, 170, 186, 187, 189, 191, 196, 212
   billiards, 51, 189, 191, 192, 193
   bowling, 51, 115, 122, 185, 187, 190,

Sports, bowling, *cont.*
        192, 193, 194, 196, 197
        206, 214, 222
  boxing, 85, 187
  coaching, 59
  conditioning, 34, 38
  croquet, 193, 214
  discus, 191, 192, 197
  exercise, 6, 12, 34, 38, 193, 195, 212, 214
  fishing, 186
  five animals, 7
  football, 50, 87, 115, 192, 196, 197, 212
    prohibitions, 9
  golf, 83, 84, 187, 188, 189, 191, 192, 193, 194, 196, 198, 212, 214
    prohibitions, 9
  gymnastics, 6, 206
  hockey, 184
  horse racing, 96, 162
    handicap match, 23
  horseback riding, 58
  horseshoes, 187, 188, 191, 192, 193, 194
  pole vault, 192
  running, 197
  shooting:
    skeet, 191
  smoker, 93
  soccer, 194, 195, 198
  softball, 187, 188, 191
  team, 205
  tennis, 58, 183, 185, 187, 188, 189, 190, 191, 192, 195, 197
  track, 196
    high jump, 191
    shotput, 188, 191
    viewing, 115, 232

Sports, *cont.*
  volleyball, 187, 189, 190, 220
  weight lifting, 194
  wheelchair, 14, 15, 73
  wrestling, 195, 206
Stadium, 5
Swimming, 55, 58, 59, 87, 122, 123, 174, 175, 187, 188, 189, 190, 191, 192, 193, 194, 195, 196, 197, 212, 213, 214, 226, 232
  diving, 195, 197

Talking, 55, 58
Television:
  viewing, 55, 59, 115, 164, 204, 207, 232
Theater (*see also* Excursions), 5, 13, 17, 58, 84, 93, 96, 102, 162, 165, 169, 175, 210, 213
  circus, 6
  comedy, 5
    musical, 17
  dramatics, 6, 214, 223
  excursions, 56
  groups, 17
  ice show, 6
  play reading group, 91
  rodeo, 16
  tape-recorded plays, 90
Toys, 4, 8, 45, 89, 214
Trampoline, 197
Travel, 115
Tumbling, 194, 196

Vacations (*see* Excursions)

Walking, 5, 55, 164, 197
Writing, 183, 185
  newspaper, 220

General Index

Activity Analysis:
  sensory-motor, 182
Adaptive behavioral levels, 202
Administration:
  finance, 125, 126
  hospital responsibility, 8
  of therapeutic recreation service, 63, 64
  sanction of, 107
  variables in program planning, 118
Affective domain, 203, 204, 205, 206, 207, 208, 209
Age:
  chronological, 111
Aging (*see* Age, chronological)
  case, 56, 228, 229
  effects upon health of, 8
  service to, 15
Amputation:
  case, 59, 87
Arthritis:
  classification system, 200

Behavioral:
  change, 82
  domains, (*see* Affective domain, 111, Cognitive domain, Sensory-motor domain)
    classification of skills in, 210, 211

Behavioral, *cont.*
  levels, adaptive, 202
  problems:
    adult, 206, 207
Blind, service to, 13
Boredom, effects of, 121
Brainstorming, 140

Cardiac disease classification system, 198, 199
Case:
  adolescent:
    center:
      mental retardation, 61, 221, 222, 225, 226
    clinic:
      hemophilia, 86
    corrections:
      second offender, 93
    homecare:
      cerebral palsy, 232
    school:
      deaf, 82
  adult:
    center:
      diagnostic, 82
    home-nursing:
      new admission, 219

General Index

Case, adult, *cont.*
    visual impairment, 93
    home-residential:
      aging, 56
      depressed, 219
    homecare:
      evaluation, 57, 88
    hospital, 54, 60
      acute anxiety, 90
      amputation, 87
      bilateral amputee, 59
      conversion reaction, 90
      depression, 89, 90
      dermatitis, 89
      emphysema, 215, 216
      evaluation, 231
      gi disturbance, 233
      hip fracture, 228, 229
      hypertension, 224, 225
      neurological, 89
      neurological (Ms), 216, 217, 218
      organic brain damage, 90
      orthopedic, 89
      plastic surgery, 89
      pleural effusion, 91
      post-operative, 89
    noninstitutionalized:
      depression, 2
      surgery, 7
    psychiatric:
      aggressive, 204, 205
      behavioral problems, 206, 207
      obsessive, 205, 206
      passive dependent, 204
      predischarge counseling, 99
      psychosis, 220, 221, 223, 226,
          227, 228
    rehabilitation:
      auto accident, 94
      quadriplegia, 98, 229, 230
    child:
      hospital:
        evaluation, 84

Cerebral palsy:
  case, 232
Classes, 161
Classification System:
  activity skills, 209, 210, 211
  arthritis, 199
  behavioral disorder, 208
  cardiac, 198

Classification System, *cont.*
  diabetes, 199
  mental retardation, 202, 203
  tuberculosis, 199
Climate:
  influence on program, 121
Clubs, 161
Cognitive domain, 200, 201, 202, 203
Committees, 161
Consultation:
  compared other roles, 67
  defined, 67
  general activities, 70, 71
  principles of, 68
  problems in, 70
Contests, 161
Convalescence, 9
Coordination:
  relationship to program, 108
Counseling:
  predischarge, 96, 97, 98
  case, 99

Deaf:
  case, 82
  service to, 13
Depression:
  case, 121, 219
  case, 2, 90
Dermatitis:
  case, 89
Diabetes:
  classification system, 200
Diagnosis, 81, 82
  case, 82
Disability (*see* Illness and Disability)
Disuse atrophy syndrome, 6
Domains, (*see* Behavioral domains)
Dynamics:
  interactive:
    inherent in activity, 162
  intragroup:
    mature interaction, 171
    premature involvement in, 171
Dysfunction:
  prevention of, 1, 2, 5, 6, 9

Educational status:
  influencing program development, 113
Emphysema:
  case, 215, 216

General Index

Equipment:
  acquisition:
    influencing program, 107
Ethos:
  influencing program development, 112
Evaluation:
  case, 84, 88
  program, 148

Finance:
  effect on program, 125, 126

Gender:
  sexual:
    influencing program development, 112
Geographic location:
  effect on program, 121
Group dynamics, (see Dynamics)

Handicap:
  word origin, 21, 22, 23
Hemophilia:
  case, 86
Homebound:
  case, 57, 88, 232
Hypertension:
  case, 224, 225

Illness and disability:
  attributable to, 5
  cure, 7
  prevention, 8
  treatment, 2, 5
Impulse, 2
Inactivity:
  effect on patients and clients, 120
Individual differences, 81
Institution:
  census:
    effect on program, 124
  climate:
    effect, 121
  finance:
    effect on program, 125, 126
  location:
    effect on program, 121
  recreation manpower needs, 124, 125
  social structure:
    effect on program, 118, 119, 120, 121

Institution, cont.
  space allocation:
    effect on program, 122
  time allocation:
    effect on program, 122, 123, 124
  total:
    concept of, 119
Intellect:
  structure of, 200
Interactive process, 162
Interest and skill:
  influencing program development, 116
Interest groups, 161
Interviewing, 83, 162
Intragroup process:
  premature involvement:
    dynamics of, 171

Kinesiological analysis, 177
  example of, 178, 179, 180, 181, 182

Leadership, 107, 132, 133, 156, 157, 158, 159
Leagues, 161
Life:
  situation altered, 94
  sustaining of, 1
Life styles:
  influencing program development, 114, 115, 116
Limitations:
  imposed by disability, 72
Loneliness:
  effect on patients and clients, 121
Lounge program, 160

Malpractice:
  medical, 4
Mental disorder:
  anxiety:
    case, 90
  classification of behavior, 208
  depression:
    case, 2, 89, 90
  historic treatment of, 6
  treatment of, 12
Mental retardation:
  case, 61, 221, 222, 225, 226
  classification system, 202, 203
  service to, 14
  treatment of, 12

Models:
    for programming, 108, 109

Needs:
    gratification of, 1
    of participants, 109, 110, 111
    recreation manpower:
        institutional, 124, 125
Neurological:
    case, 89, 90, 216, 217, 218

Objectives:
    activity, 174
    sources for preparation of, 154
    therapeutic recreation service:
        example of, 138
Observation, 82, 84
Orthopedic:
    case, 89, 228, 229

Participants:
    nature of, 109
Participation:
    abilities and skills required for, 209
Pathological play (see Play, pathological)
Pathology:
    treatment of, 1
Person:
    convalescent sick, 5
    homebound, 100
    independent, 103
    isolated, 100
    limited, 102
    needs of, 109, 110, 111
    secluded, 101
Personality:
    healthy aspects of, 81
Philosophy, 25, 43, 44
    work-play-jack, 2
Physical movements:
    classification of, 177
    fundamental, 177, 178
Play:
    pathological, 208, 209
Post-operative:
    case, 89
Prevention:
    of dysfunction, 1, 2, 5, 6, 9
    of illness, 8
Program:
    activity, 80
        elements of, 174, 175, 176

Program, *cont.*
    arthritis classification, 200
    cardiac classification, 198, 199
    content:
        bibliographic examples for, 212, 213, 214
    defined, 105
    design, 144, 145, 146
    development:
        variables influencing, 107, 108
    diabetes classification, 200
    evaluation, 148
    guidelines for, 106, 107
    implementation, 148, 149
    inherent interactive process, 162
    mental disorder:
        classification of behavior, 208
    mental retardation classification, 202, 203
    methods, 108, 109, 142, 143
    models, 108, 109
    skills:
        coding scheme for, 209
    social structures, 160
    systems analysis methods, 136
    systems analysis procedures:
        application, 137
    tuberculosis classification, 199
    variables:
        influencing development, 107, 108, 111, 112, 113, 114, 115, 116, 117, 118
Psychosis:
    case, 220, 221, 223, 226, 227, 228

Quadriplegia:
    case, 98, 229, 230

Reactive depression, 2
Recreation:
    as treatment, 5, 10, 19, 86
    behavioral dynamics of, 45, 46
    conscious use of, 10
    counseling, 57
    denied, 9
        psychodynamics of, 2
    in care plans, 86
    nature of, 1
    pathology:
        and, 20, 21
    patterns, 83
    philosophy of, 25, 43, 44

General Index 253

Recreation, *cont.*
  preventive context, 2
  service elements, 51, 52, 53
  social institutional context, 47, 48, 49
        50
  style, 83, 84
  time allocation for, 122, 123, 124
  value of, 1, 10
Rehabilitation:
  activity analysis for, 182
Research (*see* Evaluation)
Roles:
  leadership, 156, 157, 158, 159
  professional, 76
  therapeutic recreation specialist, 26, 27,
        56

Sanction:
  administrative:
    influencing program, 107
Sciatica:
  treatment of, 6
Sensory-motor domain, 176
Sheltered programming, 100
Social behaviors:
  expected, 81
Social structure:
  effect on program, 118, 119, 120, 121
Social structures:
  methods of grouping patients and
        clients, 160
Socioeconomic status:
  influencing program development, 113
Space:
  effect on program, 107, 122
Special events, 124, 161, 162
Surgery, 7
  plastic:
    case, 89
Systems analysis:
  application to therapeutic recreation
        service, 150
  influence of suprasystem, 134, 135
  introduction to, 128, 129, 130
  procedures, 137, 138
  relationship to program planning, 136

Terminology, 78
Therapeutic recreation service:
  information sources, 18
  activity programming, 80
  activity structures, 160, 161, 162

Therapeutic recreation service, *cont.*
  administration of, 63, 64
  altered life situation:
    programming in, 94
  application:
    systems analysis procedure, 138, 150,
        151, 152, 153, 154
  budgeting in, 64, 65, 66
  community development in, 62
  components of the system, 132
  concept of, 2
  consultation in, 67
  diagnosis, 81, 82
  dynamics of group life, 171
  educational elements in, 54
  effect of war on, 13, 14
  elements of, 27, 132, 133
  elimination of barriers, 71
  evaluation, 81
  facility:
    modification, 73
  goals, 31
  influence of suprasystem, 135, 136
  information sources, 75, 76, 77, 78, 79
  instruction, 60
  integration of components, 133, 134
  interviewing in, 83, 162
  levels of, 24
  manpower needs, 124, 125
  matrix of, 133
  nature of the system, 131
  objectives:
    example of, 138
    sources for, 154
  predischarge counseling, 96, 97, 98
  prescription for, 19
  principles of, 24, 25, 26, 27, 54
  professional education in, 74
  progress report:
    example of, 90
  purpose of the system, 130
  reeducative care, 24
  reconstructive care, 24
  reporting:
    observations, 82, 84
    recreation patterns, 83
    recreation style, 83, 84
    signs of behavioral change, 82
  request for service, 85, 86, 87, 89, 90, 92
        215, 216, 220, 224, 227,
        228, 229, 233
  research, 74

Therapeutic recreation service, *cont.*
   resources, 61
   sheltered experience:
      programming for, 100
   supportive care, 24
   system processes, 132
Therapeutic recreation specialist:
   leadership roles, 156, 157, 158, 159
   mental set, 82
   role of, 26, 27, 56
Therapeutic vs. therapy, 19
Time:
   effect on program, 122, 123, 124
Tournaments, 161
Treatment:
   types of, 9
Treatment of:
   illness and disability:
      historical, 2, 5

Treatment of, *cont.*
   mental disorder, 6, 12
   mental retardation, 12
   pathology, 1
   sciatica, 6
Tuberculosis:
   case, 91
   classification system, 199

Variables:
   administrative, 118, 119, 120, 121, 122, 123, 124, 125, 126, 127
   influencing program development, 107, 108, 111, 112, 113, 114, 115, 116, 117, 118
Visual impairment:
   case, 93